WAHIDA CLARK PRESENTS

Hair Therapy:

Cures for Growing your Beautiful Natural Hair

Tiffany Anderson, Natural Hair Trichologist

This is a work of fiction. Names, characters, places, and incidents either are the product of the author's imagination or are used fictitiously, and any resemblance to actual persons, living or dead, business establishments, events, or locales are entirely coincidental.

Wahida Clark Presents Publishing
60 Evergreen Place
Suite 904A
East Orange, New Jersey 07018
1(866)-910-6920
www.wclarkpublishing.com

Copyright 2018 © by Tiffany Anderson
All rights reserved. This book, or parts thereof, may not be reproduced in any form without permission.

Library of Congress Cataloging-In-Publication Data:
Tiffany Anderson
Hair Therapy: Cures for Growing your Beautiful Natural Hair
ISBN 13-digit 978-1-944992-25-5 (paper)
ISBN 13-digit 978-1-944992-81-1 (ebook)
ISBN 13-digit 978-1-944992-47-7 (Hardcover)

LCCN: 2017900826

1. Natural Hair- 2. Self Help- 3. Beauty- 4. African American- Hair - 5. Health- 6. Cosmetics - 7. Hair Care

Cover design and layout by Nuance Art, LLC
Book design by NuanceArt@aCreativeNuance.com
Edited by Linda Wilson
Proofreader Rosalind Hamilton

Printed in USA

Hair Therapy Foreward
By Wahida Clark

One year ago, today, the barber shaved my Sister-Locs, and to the floor they fell.

He asked me "do you want to keep them?" I responded, "is that what people do? It's only hair."

I was surprised at the words that came out of my mouth. Because I was a big consumer of weaves, wigs, lace-fronts, cornrow braids, fat ones, small ones, box braids, micro braids, and finally I went to Sister-Locs.

The transition was something I fell in love with. Being able to run my fingers through my own hair, washing it whenever I wanted to, put it up when I want to, or just let it be. The freedom is very exhilarating. No more being constricted to a weave or wig, even just having box braids was challenging.

Not only the freedom I fell in love with but being able to nourish my hair the way I like. The vitamins and minerals that is needed to acquire a healthy head of hair was my goal, and having Sister-Locs is what allowed me to do so. I am truly #TeamNatural and #TeamBald.

If you have recently cut your hair or plan to do so, or went natural or plan to do so, it's a new beginning and you will feel like you are reconnecting to your inner self and you're your beauty.

Wahida Clark

TABLE OF CONTENTS

Journey 1

Bad Hair Day 5

Counterfeit Hairstylist 9

Nappy or Kinky 13

Color 16

American Lye 19

Edges 31

Washing 33

Products Are to Sell 35

The Importance of Steps 39

Hair Types 42

Underneath the Weave 45

Fooled by YouTube 46

Turn Down 49

The Next Steps after the Perm 52

Daily Regimen 55

Trichology 59

Water, H2O, Agua 63

Lifetime 65

Short Hair 68

Recommendations 70

Components 73

The Common Sense of Hair Loss 75

Conspiracy 78

Oxygen 80

Warning: 82

Transitioning Techniques 85

It Takes One to Know One 92

Please Don't 94

Glossary 96

I Love My Natural Hair 104

Thank you, Lord, for giving me the strength and the courage to present this project that will encourage, uplift and enlighten new and veteran naturals on their journey to understand hair care.

Beautiful Black Girl

*Beautiful black girl where have you gone
Searching for your identity amongst superficial blondes*

*Beautiful black girl don't forget you
From Harriet Tubman to Maya Angelou*

*Beautiful black girl don't give in
To processed hair temptation that burns from within*

*Beautiful black girl help me to ignore
The stares and resentment of an unnatural world*

*Beautiful black girl don't leave me
So that I too will 'blaze a trail' in history*

Tiffany Anderson

Journey

Throughout many consultations as a natural hair stylist, I have long awaited for someone to explore the truth behind natural hair care.

Scalp after scalp I give consistent factual advice about maintaining natural hair. Time after time I receive the same reply from discouraged clients: "I have never heard that before." Whenever I hear this statement, it makes me nervous about the hair industry's true motives. Since I have been a part of the hair industry for so long, my thoughts drift to one major question: Why aren't hair professionals taking advantage of the advanced training made accessible to them? This oversight or indifference by hair professionals forces clients to seek out their own hair care information. I hope these professionals aren't purposely neglecting to educate clients in hopes that the client makes no attempt to do her own hair, but relies solely on her stylist for all her hair care needs. Some clients have told me that certain hair professionals have advised: "The only way to manage your hair is with a relaxer." Instantly, the clients believe this and blindly put their faith in a chemical-based alternative instead of in natural hair care and maintenance. This belief haunts my dreams, making it hard for me to get a good night's sleep because I'm so perplexed about how I should take action against this untruth. Daily, I battle my thoughts on how I can help the industry become a more reputable source that will encourage healthy, luxurious, chemical-free hair.

In today's society, time has gotten away from us as well as our patience. We used to take the time to care for our hair, but now it seems as if we only take time to "shop" for hair. This generation has become obsessed with superficial images and less concerned about our own image. When are we going to stop trying so hard and just be us?

When I became a part of the hair industry, the main ingredient was education. Educating yourself was a key element to becoming a force in the industry. It was also a key ingredient for success. Your knowledge alone would set you apart from your peers. As I look at what the industry has evolved into, it demoralizes my spirit. It's all about who can become the biggest influencer or blogger, and get the most money from product companies while exploiting hair products that will not work on certain hair textures. Imagine how discouraging my journey is, knowing my competitors are less educated and inexperienced, especially when many of the reviewers serve as the only test subject because they have no client base whatsoever. Yet they have gained a significant amount of praise and recognition from social media. It is unsettling when clients sit in my chair dissecting my credibility. I feel alone in the industry, as if I am the only one trying to help make a difference. I may not be the only one, but I will be the first to share with you "Hair Therapy:

Cures for Growing Your Beautiful Natural Hair." Follow me as I share a lifetime of information, consultations, techniques, and testimonials.

"As you journey with me through these chapters, I want you to understand that it is one aspect to share by educating, and it is another aspect to share through experience, but it is everything to share using knowledge because it embodies both education and experience."

-Tiffany Anderson

Bad Hair Day

Bad hair days can put us in a bad space, which can lead to deflective energy. When we feel bad, we tend to deflect that energy onto other people, especially other races. When someone has made us feel uncomfortable about something that has been out of our control our entire life, it ignites a fire inside us that is hard to put out. This fire can be anger and frustration. We are angry with ourselves, angry toward family members, coworkers, and especially toward the race we hold responsible for the rejection in the first place. We have a lot of anger toward our hair, and when it does not cooperate the way we feel it should, we want to change it. If the change is not a smooth transition, or we are uncomfortable with the results, it's "Hello, Bad Hair Day." Everyone better beware. We have internalized what we think will make other people feel better, not ourselves. We fixate on hairstyles we know our natural hair cannot and will not conform to, unless it is altered or manipulated with chemicals or extension hair. We go from short to long, black to blue, in a matter of hours, depending on how we feel. That feeling is passed down from the self-deprecating thoughts about our hair that other cultures have inflicted upon us. If someone says something in reference to our hair, it ignites our negative attitude. We become extra-sensitive when asked a basic question about the many hairstyles we adorn in such a short time. We get defensive, as if it is an unrealistic question. Most people are inquisitive to learn how creative artwork can be achieved on one's head.

Some of us will transform our hair into an 'appropriate' hairstyle because we think it's the extra incentive needed to obtain a higher position in Corporate America. In the meantime, we forget about the more important issue—the difficult struggle we had to go through to get where we are as black women in Corporate America. If we had never conformed to covert "appropriate grooming rules" in the beginning, then the powers that be would've had no choice but to accept us and our natural hair.

As we transition to our supposed 'appropriate' look—playing, lying, and redefining ourselves, we do not take self-inventory of how beautiful we already are on the inside and out. We rely only on what we are going to conform to. However, as we become more comfortable within ourselves, we get tired of playing the hair game that we have played for so many years. By this point, we have either gotten better or far worse at it. Better, knowing that we are beautiful and accepting of what we were born with as Black women. Or worse, still trying to become whom we think we are 'supposed' to be. If we are at our worst, we continue to have bad hair days and deflect our self-worth onto other people.

Don't get caught up in that old self-loathing cycle of never being satisfied with how you look. I'm not saying variety is bad, but I am saying not appreciating what you currently have is not good. It's devastating to want to be something that you are not. When you feel like this, you convert that energy on to others and the pressure onto yourself. Confidence is being happy with what you are born with, believing it and rocking it. If you would invest in what is really bothering you, like taking better care of your health, your mental state, and watching your spending and eating habits and learning more about yourself, then you will begin to get rid of the image you think you have to become in order to be accepted.

"Every day our minds are being manipulated with images based on how society thinks we should look."

-Tiffany Anderson

Counterfeit Hairstylist

A counterfeit hairstylist is a name I use to refer to the stylist who takes his or her role as a hair care professional for granted. I understood early on in the game that once I decided to do hair as a professional, I would not be a counterfeit hairstylist. My dreams and goals have always been ahead of my time and budget, but I never cut corners, even when I had limited capital. I knew my ambition would take me further in the industry as a professional, and I respected the importance of: "Educate yourself in the business that you are pursuing and not simply for the money." In order to stand out, I knew I had to offer what others were not. I chose 'quality' hair care. At the time I became a part of the natural hair movement, I noticed hair care was being neglected at an all-time high. This neglect opened up a niche for me to dive right into. I wanted to give people quality service, hair care experience, and a chance to prevent the results of long-term hair abuse.

In 2001, I began exploring alternative hair care so I could assist people suffering from hair loss. I realized I had to have the knowledge (education + experience) in order to help. At the time, there were not many creative options or versatility with natural hair that we can appreciate today. Products and hairstyles were limited, and I wanted to do what my peers were not doing, yet help simultaneously.

To build a solid clientele, I had to be exceptional at this niche. Since I was not offering the traditional chemical services that most hair professionals go to school for, I set my focus on natural hair care. I didn't put emphasis on what I wasn't doing, but on what I *had* to do. I never passed up an opportunity and tried never to let one pass me up. Even when I was unable, mismanaging funds and overbooking on more occasions than one, I stayed ready at all costs. I was determined to give quality hair care service and the most valuable information that my clients had ever received—the truth about natural hair. I studied many hair products, breaking down the chemistry of natural hair versus chemically-treated hair, evaluating the curl pattern textures and how each product worked on it. I noticed that water-based products would not penetrate natural hair as well as straight hair. The product would just slide off, leaving the hair in the same condition, as if nothing was applied. When I used the crème based products on natural hair, the product would penetrate, softening and smoothing the hair cuticle, causing the natural hair to stay moist. Once I recognized the significance and benefits of this observation, I had to share. I began educating every client that sat in my chair, helping them understand the appropriate type of moisture needed to manage and maintain natural hair. I started transitioning clients from relaxed hair to natural hair in droves. Clients who have had natural hair since birth were programmed to believe they needed a relaxer to survive. I diffused every cliché ever thrown their way about their natural hair.

*"Once you get into the beauty industry, you have already decided
what's more important: to help others or to profit from others."*

-*Tiffany Anderson*

Nappy or Kinky

Nappy or Kinky is not a texture. Curly is a texture. You will not find the words "nappy" or "kinky" in any cosmetology books. Nappy or Kinky are negative words created to describe our texture and to put down our hair. When you refer to your hair as being "nappy" or "kinky," it makes you want to take drastic measures in altering your natural hair texture because it's "too nappy" or "too kinky" to deal with. It usually results in your natural texture being treated with a chemical, or something being glued or attached to the hair. Whatever the decision, we know it's covering up the "nappy" or "kinky" hair texture. When you, however, refer to your curl pattern as curly, that thought resonates differently. Your first thought is not to get *rid* of the curl but to *define* the curl or enhance it so that it's manageable.

It is important to know that the use of different terminology depicts the decisions we will make regarding our hair care. We need to know the words that give our hair life and the words that drain the life out of our hair. When referring to our crown and glory we have to be extremely careful because we have already internalized "nappy" and "kinky" as being negative. Although we have tried to address the words in a positive light, the implication has already been set and has had a significant impact on the way we see ourselves. We must realize that when we call our hair "nappy" or "kinky," it is not a compliment. This perception is sad but rings true. Trying to fix the two words is like trying to dress up a pig. A standard has already been set: "Not good enough!" Nappy or kinky makes us feel as if we need to change our appearance, as if we won't fit in unless we are not "nappy" or "kinky" anymore.

We idolize images that do not look like us. We fantasize about how our hair will look once straightened. Although we try to unwelcome these thoughts, they stick to us because we have been convicted about our hair and looks. Finally, we concur with our temptation and get a relaxer. The cold crème on the scalp feels like an Etta James concert, and she is singing "At Last," directly to your hair. But instead of singing "your love has come along," she is singing "your hair has come around." Now you are hooked on your new *un-nappy, un-kinky* hair.

Furthermore, we must channel our spirit to embrace other hair replacement methods. We do not want to become fixated on not taking care of our curly hair. We do not want to become dependent on the weave. Some people install weaves so tight that now the hair follicles won't grow back, so they only feel comfortable wearing a weave. Do not replace your curly hair with the words "nappy" or "kinky." It will only cause resentment toward your natural hair world.

You will be left wondering why you ever got a relaxer or a weave in the first place. You will not understand that it all started with two words used to make us not appreciate our hair texture. The beauty industry does not make products for "nappy" or "kinky" hair (see Hair Type chapter).

Color

Many people are deceived when it comes to hair coloring because of the different ways you can apply the color to the hair. Some are under the impression that using rinses for your coloring preference as opposed to permanent will not damage the hair. The reason it is misunderstood is because rinses go on top of the hair cuticle and does not absorb the color like permanent color does. By it going on top of the hair cuticle and not penetrating like permanent color, allows the hair color to dissolve by the number of times the hair is washed. Permanent color penetrates the hair shaft by opening the hair's cuticle and leaving a permanent color stain on the hair, which allows the hair to absorb the color permanently. In my perspective, all hair coloring methods are chemicals because it alters the natural color of your natural hair. When you alter something you must make it do something it was not originally designed to do. So that puts the hair in jeopardy, which makes the strength of the hair vulnerable to breakage.

Before you get a permanent color service, I strongly

recommend you request a skin test. The skin test is done 48 hours prior to the color service to make sure you are not allergic to any ingredients in the color. Because the scalp is skin this should always be done, but many hair professionals ignore this step completely and your hair and scalp suffer damage if someone is allergic to hair chemicals. I believe the mere existence of a skin test is enough to reconsider the coloring process altogether.

Some people also believe that permanent color is more harmful than the semis or rinses because a skin test is not required for the other types of hair coloring, only for permanent color. In my opinion, the level of a chemical does not matter. A chemical is a chemical because it is an ingredient in the color that permits the hair color to change temporary or permanently. People have also been known to have allergic reactions to rinses, and even to a natural plant called henna that is used to permanently color the hair and temporarily tattoo the skin.

Henna is a flowering plant. The leaves of the henna plant contain a natural and very effective coloring pigment, that after mixing into a paste, you can apply directly to your hair or skin for coloring.

When my clients ask about color, I simply explain that the best color is no color. If you cannot live without color, I recommend organic color because organic color uses an oil base and eliminates the ammonia in the color which is less harmful to the hair.

*"**If you sit in my chair** once a year or twelve times a year, the condition of your hair should remain healthy."*

-Tiffany Anderson

American Lye

Lye is a strongly used alkaline solution, especially of potassium hydroxide, used for washing or cleansing. When I talk about lye it is not positive. "Lye is a dangerous product that can cause harm or even death if mishandled." Lye is the main ingredient in relaxers. The lye in the relaxer straightens the hair. The reason I use the term the "American lye" is because there are companies that are allowed to market 'no lye' relaxers to consumers. There is no such thing as a 'no lye' relaxer. It may be less lye used in a relaxer but not 'no lye.' Even when the straightening process is minimal, it is still the lye that enables the hair to become temporarily straightened until it grows out. Ever since I have been a hairstylist, I have been fortunate enough to only see a lye chemical burn one time. The client was referred to me for a braided style, and she wanted me to braid over the burn. She was totally oblivious to the severity of the burn. I recommended she seek medical attention.

TIFFANY ANDERSON

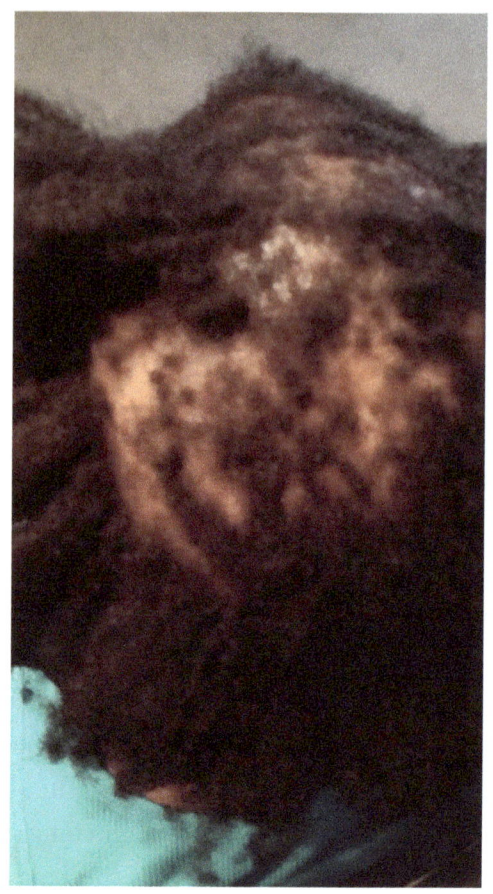

Before Trichology Services

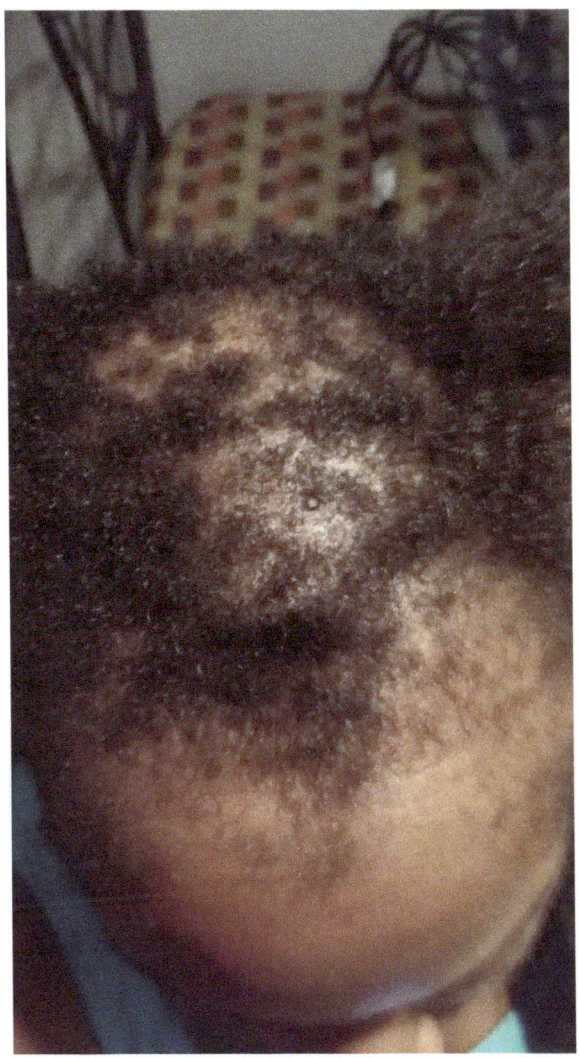

Before Trichology services were initiated by Tiffany Anderson

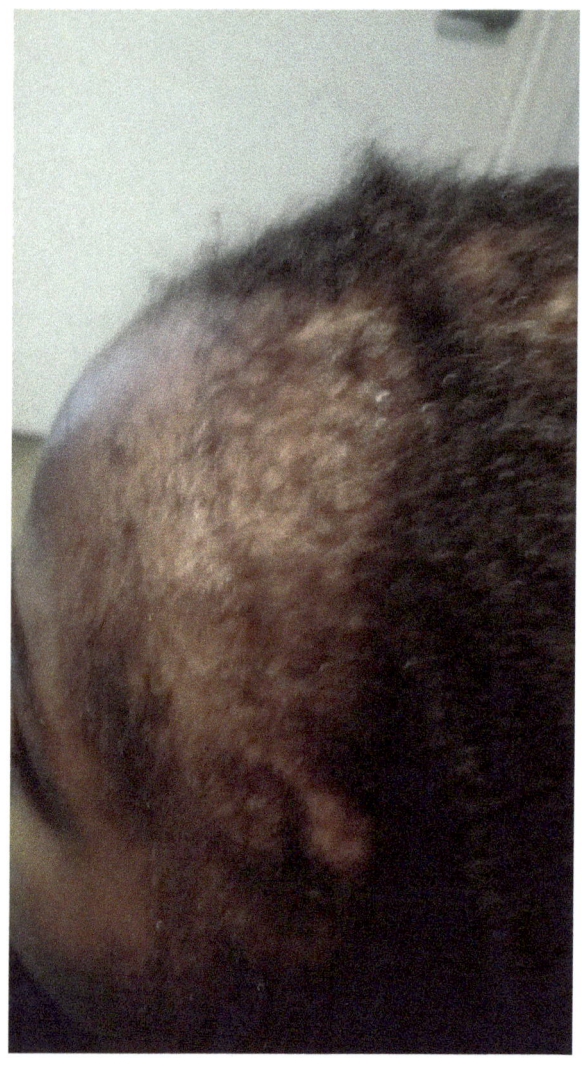

Before Trichology services were initiated by Tiffany Anderson

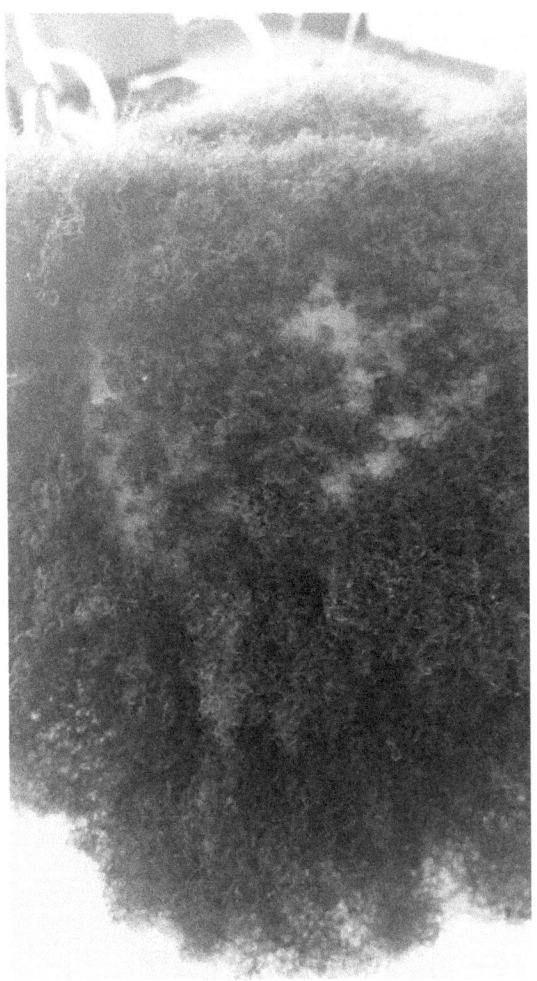

Month 1
Hair begins to grow.

Hair begins to grow in the treated areas after using Decca Plus Hair Care Line, pages (30,31,32) Decca Plus will exfoliate the scalp of excess skin and strengthen the follicles that have prevented that hair from previously coming in.

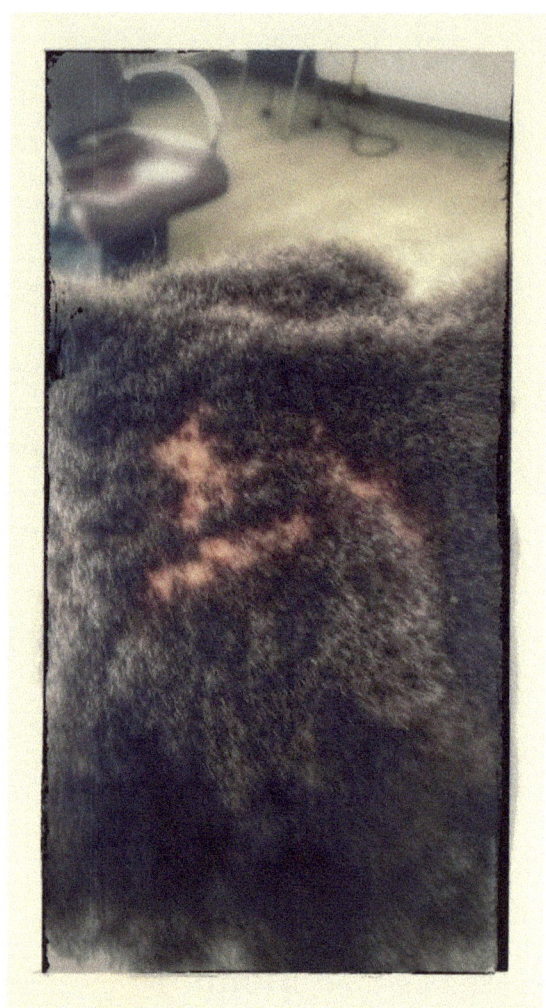

Month 2
Hair begins to fill in.

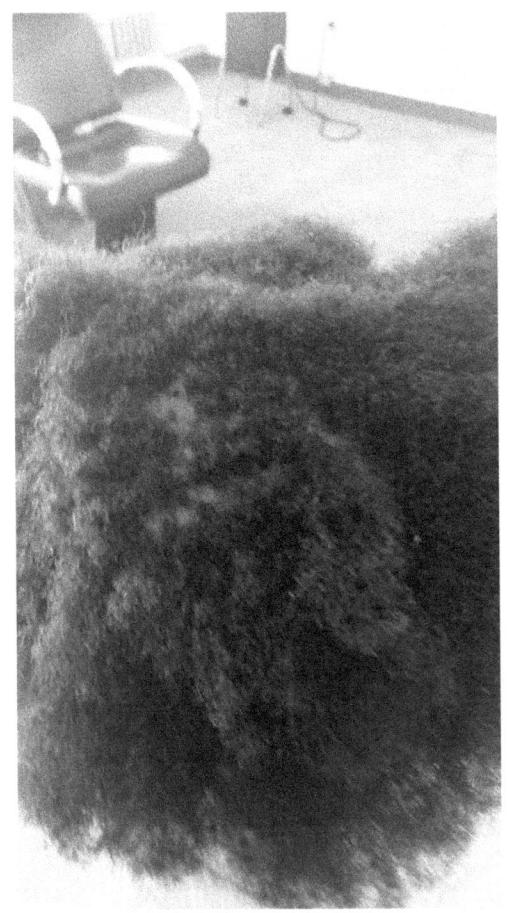

Month 2
Hair begins to fill in.
Hair is gradually filling in even more and hair follicles are beginning to restore allowing the hair to grow, pages (20,21,22)

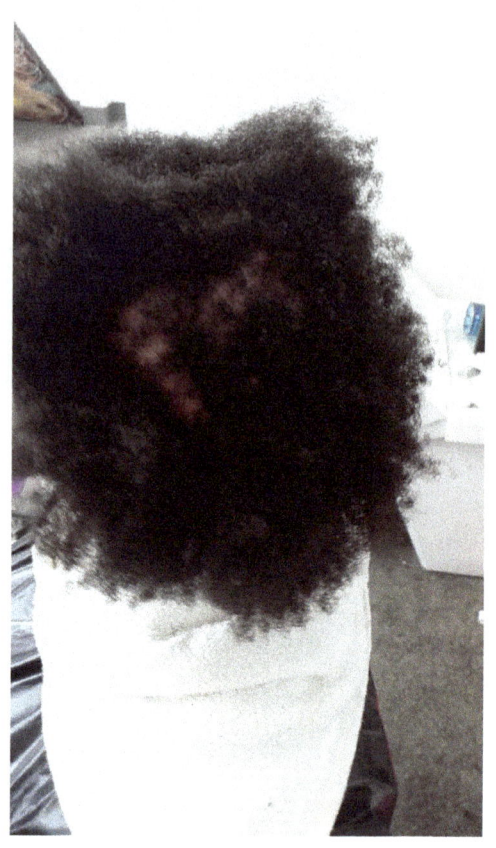

**Month 4
Hair begins to fill in.**

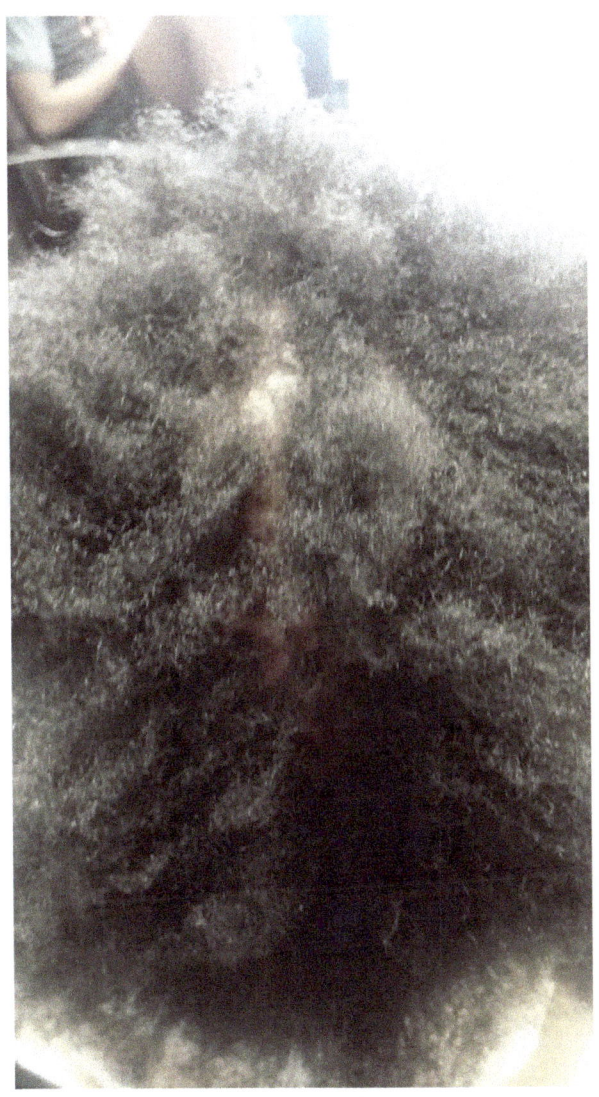

Month 8
Hair grows completely in.

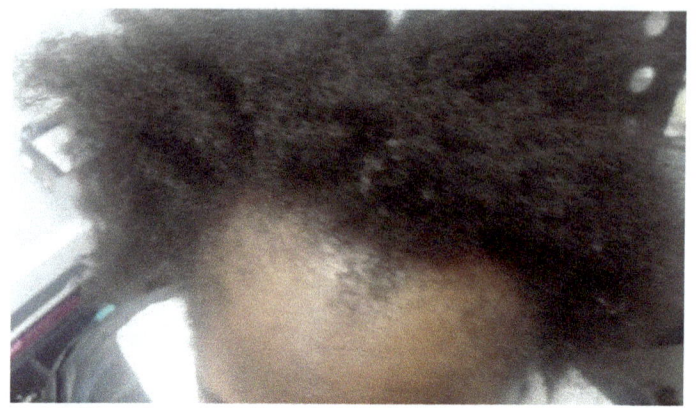

Month 8

I strongly believe it is wrong and misleading for this kind of deception to take place. I hate that we feed into the commercialized expectation of beauty. It infuriates me to know that when we look in the mirror we are not convinced we are beautiful until we have altered our image. We have disposed of our pride for relaxers and weaves. If we do not start reading the ingredients on the relaxer boxes, our hair and minds will be damaged permanently.

*"How is it the land of the free,
if we have to conform in order to be accepted?"*
- Tiffany Anderson

Edges

When you think of hair edges you should think of baby hair. That is how fragile a person's edges are. It is like a baby's hair. Baby hair is common to shed, even if nothing is being done to it. With this in mind, you should handle your edges delicately, like you would a baby's. People have no regard for how sensitive edges are, and because they don't, they take for granted how to maintain them.

Traction Alopecia is the most common sign of hair loss, and it occurs between 0 to 12 months of age. The damage can be temporary or permanent, depending on the hair follicles. This is an epidemic in the hair industry. The reason gradual hair loss is so common is because the amount of tension being applied to a baby's hairline is being ignored tremendously. This is a result of a lack of education. If you knew rubber bands cut the hair, maybe you would not use them. If you knew bumps and blisters form around hair wrapped too tight with rubber bands, maybe you would take the hair out of the rubber bands. If you knew it was okay to allow a baby's hair to be free and worn out, maybe you wouldn't pull on it as much. As you get older, the same advice must be understood. Braids, weaves, and relaxers all cause Traction Alopecia. The hair needs oxygen, and when something is too tight on the skin it will cut off the circulation. Have you ever been told as a child: "Do not put that rubber band around your wrist, or you will cut off your circulation?" Well, that happens to be true. Scalp is skin and skin is scalp. Edge education is very important when caring for natural hair because what you don't know will leave you edge-less.

Washing

Washing hair is overrated. For some reason, people think that their hair is dirty; they also feel that the more they sweat the more they need to wash their hair. Sweat is not dirt; your hair is not dirty. The more you wash your hair, the more you put your hair at risk for shedding, breakage, and also thinning. People are unaware of the harsh chemical water has in it that causes the most damage to hair. Water is sterilized with chlorine, a gaseous element which kills bacteria. It has so much of it, that it causes the water to be hard, . Chlorine also kills the natural oils and moisture our hair produces in order to sustain our healthy hair. The scalp is also compromised with the excessive use of water. The scalp becomes tight, dry, and itchy. When this happens, it will eliminate the amount of hair follicles being produced as well as kill off the hair that is already there. The more you wash the hair, the more chlorine your hair absorbs, and it becomes dry, brittle, and will break off like a dead leaf. It will also counteract against the products you are using because chlorine strips everything good out of the hair.

Chlorine is used to kill bacteria in water and that's also what it does to the hair. So the more you wash your hair, the more you are killing it, not cleansing it.

Products Are to Sell

When you think of natural hair products, you get a sense of relief that finally something has been formulated to fit your hair care needs. You think: "This is what I've been waiting on my whole life; my prayers have been answered." That is the excitement you feel, until you realize you have exhausted an entire paycheck trying to figure out which natural hair products will work for your hair type. Hoping that what the magazines and commercials promised will hold true. You can't wait to get home, anticipating the results. You read all the directions twice, and now the transformation process begins. As you go through each method step by step, it seems as if the process is taking longer than the directions suggested, but it's okay because you are in it for the long haul. You are committed to the promised results. The results that never happen! You are left disappointed, dissatisfied, and discouraged to the point that you believe there is something wrong with you, or worse, your hair. Once you manifest these thoughts and not the actual deception of the product, you become the industry's best product junkie. You buy everything the market comes out with, in search of the right product for your hair. Finally, you make the big decision to go to a natural hair stylist.

Although you are seated in the stylist's chair, you already have your mind made up that she cannot do anything for you because all the products you used have failed you. The stylist assesses your hair and your daily regimen. You listen to this information that you have never heard from a natural hair stylist, or seen on commercials, or read on the back of any products you have used before. You are skeptical of what you have just heard because you have product anxiety. You know the information is probably true, but you decide not to believe the source because you have been let down by previous hair products that claimed to deliver but never did. The stylist's knowledge and skills were not enough to convince you that it's not your hair but the ineffectiveness of the products. If you have desired manageable hair, now you can have it, if you abstain from what you have been doing that has not been working.

Think about how much money you have invested in hair products, and how full your cabinets are with unresolved hope. You don't want to go home and get rid of them because you have invested in your own mini store. What do you do? You become fearful and ignore the advice you were just given because you think the stylist is not being genuine. Many thoughts run through your brain, but none of them are: *Products are marketed toward me only with the intent to sell.* Companies will sell you a dream to sell their products, knowing the products are not going to work on any hair texture. What product companies do not share is that when products need to reach a mass market with high demand, the ingredients in the original formula has to be manipulated. This is usually done by adding water and synthetic ingredients that will do more harm over time than good. Another way companies let you know their products will not do as promised is by using models (who are allowed to wear their own hair) to advertise their product. They are selling the face, not the product.

To prevent you from being further bamboozled, I now refer to different hair products according to grades (Grade A thru Grade D). Grade A products are professional products and are only acquired through local salons or a beauty supply that requires the purchaser to be licensed. This is because the ingredients in these products are less likely to be manipulated, and the potency is consistent with the original formula. Therefore, the hair benefits more and not the company's pockets. Grade B products are homemade. They are created to offset the products that contain mostly water, parabens, and alcohol. We don't necessarily know if they will work, but we do know that they will not damage the hair. Grade C products are products a beauty supply can sell and call professional, making it seem as though the products being sold are not as diluted. Grade D products are the lowest grade in my book. They are the products being sold in box stores. These products are formulated strictly to sell in quantity. The manufacturers behind such products do not care if they will work. They are the most diluted and are only used for selling purposes, not for results.

"Natural hair has nothing to do with confidence and everything to do with appreciation."

-Tiffany Anderson

The Importance of Steps

According to the Bible, things are to be done in order. Meaning, the arrangement or disposition of people or things, in relation to each other, should be according to a particular sequence, pattern, or method. When it comes to hair care, we need to associate the same order. Steps two and three are just as important as step one. There are several steps to shampooing the hair. When you understand the reason behind steps two and three, you will not disassociate it from the process.

Shampooing cleanses the hair from dirt and build up, washing out the hair's natural oils and moisture. This should be done with a sulfate-free clarifying shampoo. After the hair is shampooed, it feels hard because the cuticles are infrared. In order to smooth out the hair's cuticles, it needs to be washed one time with a hydrating or moisturizing shampoo. This will restore the hair's natural oils and moisture. Once the moisturizing shampoo is rinsed out, the hair needs to be deep conditioned. A deep conditioner is when the hair is conditioned with heat and a conditioning cap. The heat allows the conditioner to penetrate the hair cuticle deeper, and the cap prevents the hair from drying out. The conditioner will also start the moisturizing process, bringing the hair's pH level down and smoothing the hair's cuticle so the hair will be soft once the conditioner is rinsed out. After the conditioning process has been completed, you must use a leave-in conditioner to moisturize the hair as the hair begins to dry. The leave-in conditioner stays in the hair, sealing the hair's cuticle so it will not dry out as it begins to dry, and it acts as a heat protector if heat is used. When leave-in conditioner is applied, you will separate the hair either by finger separating or by using a wide-tooth comb. Sections may vary depending on hair density. You may coil-twist the hair and let it air dry, or blow dry each section. If any of these steps are neglected, over time the hair will not promote growth and will reveal dryness and breakage.

"I am obligated to tell the truth about hair care; I am not obligated to product companies that embellish the truth."

-Tiffany Anderson

Hair Types

Do not be concerned about which hair type you have. Products are made for textures *not* types. Curly, straight, wavy are all hair textures not hair *types*. This is very misleading to new naturals, and it draws people into purchasing products from inexperienced people and the companies that create and sell them. There is really no such thing as "hair type." It is irrelevant and very confusing. What you must understand is that having a curly hair texture may consist of coarse curly, medium curly, or fine curly. Your Trichologist should be able to assist you in purchasing Grade A products. This will eliminate the disappointment of trying to figure out which type you may or may not be. Hair texture does not change, but you can have different textures on one head. For example, your hair can be curly fine around the perimeter of your head and curly coarse in the center of your head. This is very common and will determine how a style is achieved. The density of your hair impacts how much product you need to apply. For instance, if you have thick coarse hair, you will apply more product to your hair than if your hair is fine and shallow.

Density is the compactness of a substance (it refers to the thickness). There are several types of textures: straight, curly, and wavy. These textures can have different densities, such as fine to thick. Even with different textures, you should not have to use multiple products to add moisture to your hair. You should know that curly hair requires a lot of moisture to smooth and relax the cuticle because of the hair's coiled state. Moisture penetrates better than oil because the molecule in oil is too large. Now if you have fine curly hair, it may seem as though the oil is penetrating, but that is because fine curly strands are smaller than the strands on coarse curly hair. When dealing with straight hair you will not need to apply a lot of moisture, because you don't want your hair weighed down, and straight hair will hold the moisture because the cuticle is smooth.

"We treat our hair the way people have made us feel about our hair."

-Tiffany Anderson

Underneath the Weave

In order to tackle what's underneath the weave, we have to understand that, that is where it all started. Underneath the weave is our original pallet, our crown and glory. To me, we have to make sense of what goes on underneath the weave.

Underneath the weave, hair is growing. For hair to grow it needs to be stimulated. Underneath the weave is a scalp. Scalp is skin, and if the skin's circulation is cut off, the hair will fall out. Underneath the weave are hair follicles. Hair follicles are the root of the hair. Underneath the weave is skin.

Fooled by YouTube

Don't be fooled by YouTube! YouTubers grab your attention in the same fashion that product companies do to entice you to buy their products. This can result in you becoming fooled by the outcome of a style. When you are unaware of what to look for when it comes to styling your hair, you may be deceived by the appearance of the style. This happens quite often on YouTube. People are becoming obsessed with different style techniques that can be done, but are overlooking the process of *how* it's being done. If you have taken the time to grow your natural hair out, surely you do not want to pull out what you have grown for one cute style on YouTube. To avoid this from happening, do not attempt the styles on your own. Some YouTubers are professionals and experienced, so they know what they are doing. Find an experienced hairstylist who is invested in healthy hair care. Ask to see photos of their work and testimonials. Ask about the process that will be taking place to achieve the style. If they only seem consumed with the style, continue to look elsewhere. YouTubers like to present that every hair technique is a DIY job that can be created by an inexperienced person, and that is not the case. Do not be a YouTube victim, manipulated and deceived by the trick of the camera. The deception is real, and it's challenging for a professional like myself with decades of experience and results, to reach a YouTube follower. That client's loyalty is with the YouTube channel. People value the amount of subscribers instead of true knowledge. At the end of the day it's the solutions that matter, not concepts that may or may not work.

*"We take our insecurities out on our hair.
If we are feeling bad, we want a new hairdo."*
                                         -Tiffany Anderson

Turn Down

In this era, it seems as if the phrase 'turn up' has infected hairstylists. They have no affection for a person's natural hair, but all the love is poured into a weave. I can remember when ladies didn't want you to know they even wore a weave. My, how times have changed! I am aware of how fun weaves are and how exciting it is to change into a new look at the drop of your dime. My concern is the miseducation. There are people who suffer from permanent baldness and alopecia and they get a weave to cover up the damage. Most times, the damage is caused by the weaves in the first place. Don't offer me a weave if I came in for a natural hairstyle, and then say that this is a protective style for my natural hair. This mentality has been going on for a long time. A client with natural hair goes in for a press and curl but comes out with a relaxer. Give the client what she requested, or tell her how she can achieve it without a weave or chemicals.

Today there is no reason for the client or stylist to be uninformed about caring for natural hair. Stylists can take advanced training courses which have always been available. That's if they choose to invest in expanding their knowledge. When you offer someone something they don't need or didn't ask for, the implication is that they need more to be happy. For example: "I need straight hair or extensions to feel fierce and beautiful." People want to be told the truth about their hair. We should listen to the needs of our clients and not the needs of our pocketbooks. I challenge the hair industry to "turn down" and stop selling unrealistic dreams and teach people how to take care of their own hair. That way they will begin to appreciate what they have and will pass on the pride to their children, the power to their nieces, and the progress to their granddaughters. When you say you are proud of who you are, yet still cover up your pride, it contradicts what you say. Don't put out the wrong message. Don't be ashamed of your crown and glory!

"It is okay to compliment my natural hair instead of staring at it."

-Tiffany Anderson

The Next Steps after the Perm

It is very scary to transition from relaxer to natural. We don't know how we are going to wear our natural hair, nor are we familiar with the upkeep involved to maintain natural hair. In order to move forward with the process, we must understand the difference so our expectations are not confused. Keep in mind that natural and relaxed hair are two different textures. Relaxed hair is natural hair that has been chemically altered, leaving the hair permanently straight until it is grown out. Natural hair is non-chemically treated curly hair that coils, shrinks, and comes in several textures (coarse, fine, or medium). Many people are unaware of how their natural hair feels, or what it can or will not do once unrelaxed. This is because it has been relaxed for so many years and for so many reasons. The main reason is for so long someone has suggested that natural hair is bad, and it will not be accepted. As we have evolved, we have gotten rid of that stereotype to a certain degree. Now we have come full circle to the next steps after the *perm*.

There are two ways to embrace your natural hair transition. The first way is to cut all of your natural hair off in one haircut; this has been called the "big chop." The second is to gradually trim your hair as it grows out until all of the relaxer has been trimmed off. Both processes take about six to twelve months to give you at least six inches of new growth to work with. After you make the decision to begin your natural hair journey, you need to understand that the products you used for your relaxed hair will not be used on your natural hair. Relaxed hair products are usually water-based products that give permed hair lots of movement called "body." With natural hair, you want it to hold its shape and be manageable, so you use moisture-based products. The products containing moisture will penetrate the cuticle more thoroughly in curly hair, leaving it soft and manageable. If you use water-based products on natural hair, it will not penetrate the hair's cuticle and will slide off, leaving the hair dry and brittle.

The next step is having the right tools to use on your natural hair. The tools will be:

1. Grade A Decca shampoo and conditioner that will cleanse and restore the hair's health.

2. A wide-tooth comb to detangle the hair.

3. Duck bill and butterfly clips will keep the hair separated while styling or moisturizing and prevent strand snagging.

4. A shower cap, a satin sleep cap, and a scarf to hold the hair's natural moisture in when showering and

sleeping.

Next, you need to choose styles that will not jeopardize the integrity of your hair. Last, you need a good daily regimen (See next chapter *Daily Regimen*).

Daily Regimen

A plan or a regulated course, such as a diet, exercise, or treatment that is designed to give a good result.

Most people associate shedding, thinning, balding, and itching with age and heredity. A person's daily regimen is never taken into consideration. What you do every day can change the course of hair loss. For example, the causes of diabetes can be associated with a poor diet and heredity, but establishing a daily routine such as eating healthy and exercising can minimize or eradicate it. Many times, if you change these behaviors, you can prevent or reverse the progression, eliminating the disease all together. Like any disease, hair will also give you signs that it is not well, such as shedding, thinning, balding, and itching. These symptoms are warning signs to discontinue what you are doing, otherwise the progression of the symptoms will continue. We tend to ignore the signs because we are programmed to think that hair loss is due to age or heredity. We do not think that excessive itching can be caused by the scalp drying out from how often we use water on the hair. We forget that water rinses not penetrates the hair cuticle. So every time we use H2o, we are rinsing off natural oils developed in the hair to create natural moisture needed to make the hair cuticle strong. Once the hair is strong, it is less likely to break off, shed, or thin.

When you think of chlorine, you think of swimming. How easy it is to forget that chlorine is used in our faucet water, the same faucet water that we drink and cook with as well as wash our hair in. **Chlorine is used as a bleach, oxidizing agent, and disinfectant in water purification.** Imagine using water daily or weekly thinking you are adding moisture to the hair. Your results will be an overly dry scalp and excessive itching, an obvious sign to change your daily regimen by eliminating water from your daily routine.

We know that thinning comes before balding. No one goes to sleep then wakes up bald one day. Majority of the time there are signs, and the most common sign is thinning. Most males wash their hair everyday with the cheapest shampoo or soap, never conditioning, never moisturizing, just washing out all of the natural nutrients that benefit the hair. Imagine doing this from a preteen until you are in your mid-twenties, early thirties. I would say that you should be thinning, possibly even balding. But you ignore the obvious signs and doubt your contribution to the gradual hair loss. Because your father or grandfather had the same regimen, you think the thinning and balding is hereditary. You continue this behavior until the hair screams off the head completely, or horseshoes into male or female pattern baldness. Individuals will have a greater chance at preventing hair loss if they do not ignore the signs or symptoms. Changing your daily regimen can be scary because if you stop what you are doing, you may make the hair come off faster or you may stop it. Either way it's a 50/50 chance, so what do you do? You go for what you know and continue the same behavior to melt your hair away permanently.

TESTIMONIAL

"My hair was extremely dry, thin, and falling out. I was at my wits' end until I met Tiffany at Tiffany's Natural. Tiffany's recommendations to cut my damaged ends, apply daily moisture, massage my scalp and protect, nurture, and love my hair was the prescription I needed to bring about positive change. After committing to her recommendations and two months of hair and scalp treatments, I see amazing results. I now have new hair growth, healthier hair and scalp. I am loving my natural hair and the versatility of styles by Tiffany. Tiffany is truly a gifted and talented hair care professional that has restored my hair and scalp. Thank you! Thank you! Thank you!"

-Claudia N

Trichology

Trichology is the study of hair and scalp disorders. The focus is on the condition and health of the hair and scalp. Trichology does not treat symptoms but investigates the cause of the problem and recommends products that are customized to treat each specific disorder. The services are aligned for each client individually, whether it be a cancer survivor, a person suffering from alopecia, chemical damage, or thinning. Trichology caters to a wide spectrum of hair and scalp disorders. Most dermatologists treat topical symptoms such as fungus and eczema. The products they administer are for that purpose, not hair care disorders. The ingredients in the products that trichologists use play a major part in helping the hair reach the maximum benefits. A trichologist will monitor the progression of the client's hair and scalp to ensure the products are yielding results. Then the trichologist will incorporate a healthy daily regimen that the client agrees to before the client's next visit.

There are many different forms of alopecia, but the most common is Traction Alopecia, caused by tension which occurs in the first months of birth. This is due to putting too much stress on a hairline by using rubber bands and hair knockers. When this is done repeatedly it becomes excessive, and anything done excessively can cause permanent damage, which leads to traction alopecia and a receding hairline. Another common form is alopecia areata, caused by the skin being chemically burned from relaxers. Those suffering from alopecia areata experience hair loss in various places where the scalp has been damaged. The scalp will appear discolored with light or darker spots. If it is white, there is a possibility the hair may never come back. If it is brown, there is a possibility it may come back by exfoliating the scalp (removing some layers of dead skin that may prevent the hair from pushing through). A healthy scalp is flesh colored. Most of these forms can be prevented if you change your hair care behavior. A relevant way to start reversing signs is to completely eliminate the amount of tension you are putting on the hair. Stop using all chemicals, limit how often you use water to once a month, avoid using shampoos that contain negative parabens and sulfates. You should use scalp cleansing products by Decca.

    The photos below show before and after images of clients who have undergone trichology treatments:

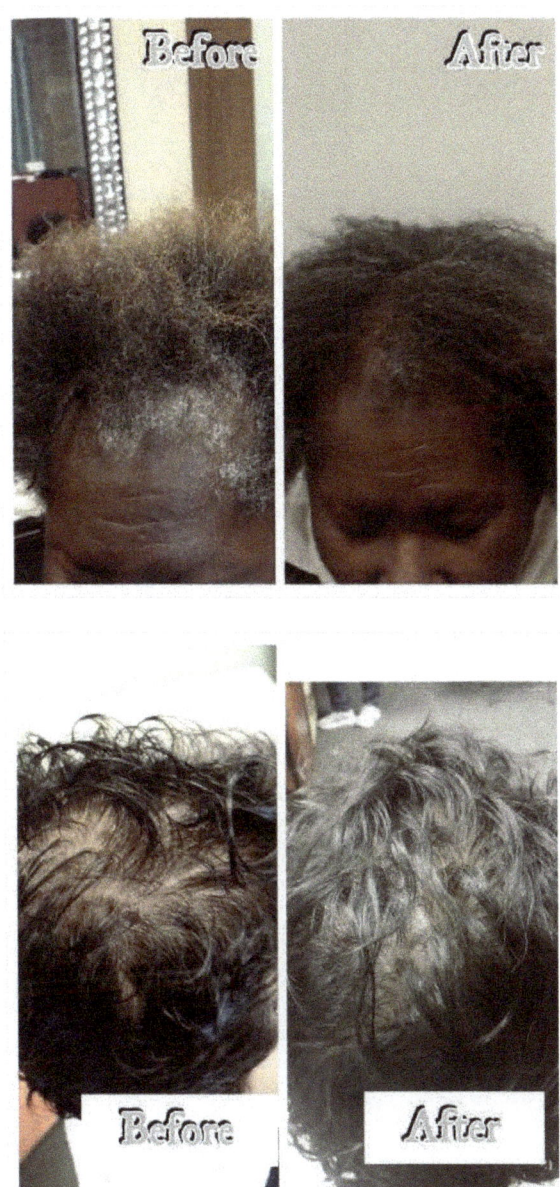

"Most people disassociate scalp from skin and ignore the warning signs on relaxer boxes that state: wear gloves, do not come in contact with the skin. Yet they are still applied to the scalp every day."

-Tiffany Anderson

Water, H2O, Agua

Water has a misrepresentation when it comes to its benefits to the hair. This comes from how we associate the way water replenishes the body. We assume it has the same effect on the hair, but it doesn't. When you use water on the hair, it rinses out all the natural properties needed to retain the hair's natural moisture and nutrients. Think about after a bath how dry your skin becomes if you do not moisturize. The skin will dry out, chafe, and itch. In retrospect, the hair will do the same from dehydration, become dry and brittle and the scalp will itch and the hair will break off. Water will do the same to the hair because it is on the outside not the inside. If you consider what water does to the body; it cleanses and rinses as well. We drink water to flush out the junk we have consumed. You use water to rinse off the product you have saturated your hair with. I have such a hard time reaching people in regards to this issue because somewhere in their brains they are convinced that water adds moisture to the hair, which is not true.

"Six in ten (6 in 10) girls stop doing what they love because they feel bad about their looks."

-Dove

Lifetime

No matter what lifetime you are in, the most important part of hair care is and will continue to be the preparation. From the shampoo to the style, this order must be consistent. Style is at the end because it is the least important, not unimportant, because if the style is created carelessly it can damage the preparation. When you shampoo and condition correctly but braid the hair adding excessive tension, you are jeopardizing the hair and edges and have defeated the purpose of preparation. Healthy hair must be top priority. If the hair is unhealthy and is damaged or broken off, it will be difficult to accomplish a desired look. Nine times out of ten you will not be satisfied with the end results, and some stylists might suggest you add extensions to create balance, volume, or length to camouflage hair imperfections. You can avoid this type of style disappointment by not neglecting the care of natural hair. Once you allow unqualified people to recommend unhealthy styles and use Grade D products, you put your hair's potential at risk. To eliminate hair disappointment by a stylist, you can start by asking one basic question: What products do you use?

If a stylist does not tell you a professional brand of products they use, I would question their expertise. If they do not tell you why you need to use a specific product and what it will prevent, I would question their experience. If you go in for a specific request, and they persuade you to do something else that will damage the hair, they are unqualified. A qualified stylist will recommend that you see someone else when they notice something is out of their scope. They will not try to cover it up or fix it. They will not lead you to believe your hair will do something that it cannot do. Qualified people should have their own before and after photos and testimonials of their own work from satisfied clients.

"I do the best I can with the hair I have to work with."
-Tiffany Anderson

Short Hair

When you have short hair or are bald, people often think there is no hair maintenance involved. I explain that when it comes to hair and scalp there is no such thing as 'no maintenance,' only low maintenance. The maintenance in caring for short hair or a bald head may not include having to braid or twist the hair daily, but it will always include a healthy daily regimen using Decca Plus hair care products. As long as you have a scalp you must make sure it is healthy. Decca Products will ensure that your scalp is not being neglected from the proper moisture and conditioning it needs by the ingredients it is formulated with.

    These products also work in stimulating the scalp, which is very important when it comes to blood circulation. Once the scalp is stimulated consistently, it will continue to promote healthy hair growth. Stimulation can be done by massaging the scalp, brushing it, or by using moist heat from hair dryers or steam. When the scalp is being stimulated using moist heat, the heat opens the hair follicles and pores, purifying the scalp of toxins within. When the scalp is being stimulated with a brush, the boar bristles exfoliate the skin as well as stimulate it.

Anytime you create stimulation to the scalp you increase circulation.

Recommendations

When clients come to me they want to know how good I can make their hair look. They are reluctant to hear what is best for their current hair situation. For example, if I tell someone they should get a particular style, they are all in, no questions asked. But if I tell them what they need to do to get their hair in a good healthy condition, they ask a ton of questions, reluctant to hear my expertise. People do not believe #hairgoals are achievable when they take on the required steps to care for their hair. I know this experience sounds all too familiar to doctors who tell their patients to lose weight by eating right, but they don't want to hear that. They want to hear what will make them feel better instantly instead of understanding that losing 20 to 50 pounds will enhance their well-being on the inside and outside. The same concept is consistent when it comes to hair care. Don't allow your mind to be blurred by unrealistic images that are being presented to you. When the doctor or trichologist advises you on what you need to do, the sooner you begin the process, the faster you will see the results you have been longing for. If you want natural hair and you have a relaxer, commit to not getting a relaxer anymore. Or, if you are really bold, cut the relaxer out. Change begins in the mind first, so change your mind and you will receive different results. You have to make a conscious decision to commit to changing your hair care behaviors in order to reach your full hair growth potential.

"Listen to what needs to happen to your hair instead of what you want to happen to your hair."

-Tiffany Anderson

Components

Components are made up of important elements that we need to survive or grow. The body needs oxygen, water, food, shelter, and sleep to survive. A plant needs water, air, nutrients, and sunlight to grow. The hair needs oxygen, stimulation, and moisture to grow. If these components are interrupted, the hair's life structure is compromised.

"You can have all the ingredients, but without the recipe the components will not blend together."

-Tiffany Anderson

The Common Sense of Hair Loss

I was told many years ago that common sense was not common to some people. This rings true when it comes to the science of hair. In my world there is not much science, but more common sense to hair growth. Hair has a domino effect, starting with the care of it. If you wet or wash your hair every day, the effect you are going to get is dry, brittle hair. If you use chemicals on your hair, over time your hair will thin and start to bald. You do not have to be a rocket scientist to understand certainty. The people I see on a daily want their hair back. Some people even bring me photographs of how their virgin hair was before it started falling out, which is before they began doing it themselves. People want their virgin hair back, but are still invested in chemicals and weaves. Yes, you heard me correct. Chemicals! I ask the question: "Is this common sense or science?" As I consult with this customer, I contemplate charging for this common sense information. Recently, I received an email from a mentor offering a new procedure for hair loss called platelet rich plasma hair restoration (PRP). Stem cells from one part of the body are transplanted directly into the pore performing follicles to stimulate new hair growth. Sounds fancy enough to work, right? Please! The model for this procedure has bleached blonde permed hair. She has her high school picture displaying her non chemical-treated virgin hair that is full and healthy and she wants that back. This client has been manipulated to think this procedure will give her, her thick, full head of hair back. In order to get back something you had, you have to stop what you have been doing to create the problem in the first place. That begins with changing your daily regimen. If you are accustomed to engaging in an unhealthy daily hair regimen, no matter what procedure you get, the results are going to continue to be the same. You have to change your hair behavior by not succumbing to what generated the hair loss in the first place.

"You will not find the words "Kinky" and "Nappy" in a cosmetology dictionary, but we still use those words in reference to our hair."

-Tiffany Anderson

Conspiracy

For all the reasons people use chemicals on their hair, they should have the same amount of reasons for not using chemicals on their hair. I have addressed how chemicals damage the hair and scalp, but we do not take into consideration the amount of time we are inhaling and breathing in those same chemicals that are breaking down the hair's natural fiber and bonds. What is it breaking down on the inside while we are inhaling them? If a product is so potent that it requires you to wear gloves to apply it, maybe you should use a mask also, as if you are in a chemist's lab, or better yet, stay away from it altogether.

Most black women spend majority of their time in a salon where chemicals are being used and inhaled all day. Did you know there is a 20% higher death rate in African American women than in White women with cancer? Sure we can associate this to late detection and obesity, but we also need to take into consideration the excessiveness of our beauty regimen. We are the only race that will indulge so eagerly in the consumer market. The faster they say a product will work, the faster we are at the store trying to achieve the swiftness of the effect. Not understanding that the faster something does work usually comes at a price. In the consumer market, the price is your health. You will get those instant benefits, but you will also get a list of discomfort and wonder why you're feeling so bad but look so good. If something is faster, it is because something artificial is making it faster. We have to accept that cosmetology is the use of chemicals. This is why there are not many ethnic styles in the study of cosmetology. Most communicable diseases can be transferred through cosmetology services. That is why sanitation is at the forefront of cosmetology. Just think about who benefits the most from becoming a cosmetologist. You have to go to school, obtain a license, and pay taxes. When we do our own hair and embrace our own culture we benefit the most by passing on our traditions to our children and grandchildren. If we become distracted and focus on how the world wants us to look, we will continue to send out the wrong message that something is wrong with the way we look. And nothing is wrong with the way we look; it's the way we think that needs to be altered.

Oxygen

Oxygen is the lifeline between the hair and scalp. For example, if you cut off the circulation to the scalp by applying too much tension and pressure on the hair, you will suffocate the hair's follicles. They become weak and form a white bulb at the root and eventually pop off. Oftentimes you can do this one time and damage the follicles so bad that the hair will never grow back. Or you can continue this pattern over time, and the damage will progress and prevent the hair from ever growing back again. Tension can be related to a number of hair procedures we do every day, but the most common are from ponytails and braids. From the time a child has hair on their head, the amount of tension that is applied will determine the survival rate of the hair. Did you know that baby hair is called baby hair because of how soft and fragile the hair is at birth and not because the hair is on a baby? A baby's hair is going to shed naturally within the first year. This is why people are surprised when the baby's hair begins to metamorphosize from one texture to another in a short time. If you do not take the necessary precautions to prevent the hair from shedding or coming out, it will happen sooner than later.

Warning:

- Do not shampoo the baby's hair every day. I recommend once a month; same as if the child was older. Remember, these habits stay with your child throughout their life. You are their first hair trainer.
- Do not use baby shampoo sold in supermarkets. It is very harsh and will dry out the baby's hair, and it may even cause cradle cap. It acts like soap, and it does not benefit curly textured hair.
- When you shampoo the baby's hair, make sure you condition and moisturize the hair as well.
- Avoid using rubber bands because they cut the hair and cut off the circulation when pulled too tight.
- Eliminate the use of headbands because they cut off the hair's circulation if they are too tight.
- Avoid pulling the hair back if at all possible. This is when traction alopecia begins.
- Avoid putting things on top of the hair for style, like

hats. Hats suck up the natural moisture in the hair.

- Avoid using water-based products on the hair. Water-based products will gradually dry the hair out over time.

- Let the hair be free to dance as much as possible within the first year. Keep it moisturized at all times.

"Healthy hair is the best hair."
-Tiffany Anderson

Transitioning Techniques

A style can appear to be very simplistic, but without the appropriate technique, it will be unattainable. Styles should be created by an experienced professional so the health of the hair is not compromised in any way. All it takes is one time to jeopardize the hair's integrity, and it may be the last because you can damage it to where it does not grow again. One of the advantages that a professional has above a DIY stylist is that they can see what they are doing. That alone speaks for itself. A lot of women are nervous when it comes to transitioning their hair back to its natural state. This fear comes from not knowing how to manage the hair, or which styles they can wear in between as the hair grows out, if they are not interested in the big chop. I am going to share two styles that can be worn through the transitioning stage from relaxer to natural, or on straight hair and you just want something different.

The first step in attaining a particular style is supplies. If you do not have all the supplies, your hair will not turn out the way you desire it to. The supplies will help you navigate through the technique smoothly. These techniques are advanced techniques and should be done by an experienced natural hair care stylist.

Two-Strand Flat Twist Technique

Supplies: 4 butterfly clips, 4 duckbill clips, styling comb, rattail comb, leave-in conditioner, moisturizer

Step 1: Apply moisturizer to moisturize the hair and protect it from the heat.

Step 2: Apply leave-in conditioner to the hair and use as a setting lotion; the leave-in conditioner will not dry out the hair as much as the setting lotion.

Step 3: Section the hair in two sections down the middle using the butterfly and duckbill clips.

Step 4: Part the hair into pinky-sized sections starting in the middle like you are preparing to cornrow.

Step 5: Begin to two-strand twist the hair to the scalp, repeating steps 3-5 until hair is completely twisted.

Step 6: Sit under hair dryer for 1 to 2 hours or until hair is completely dry.

Step 7: After hair is dry, take out twists and style and wear as desired.

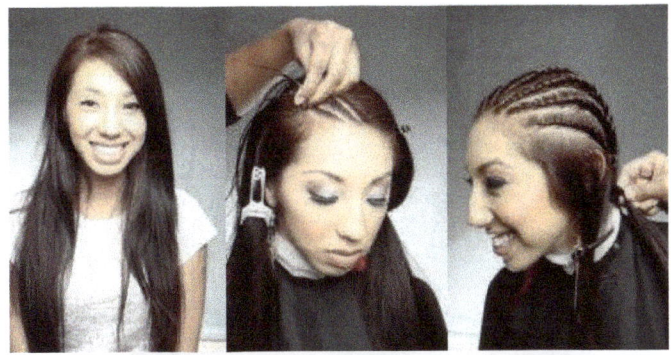
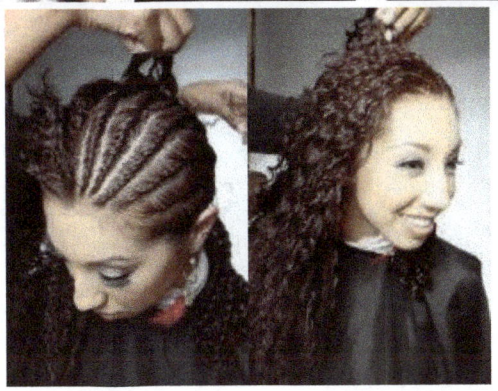

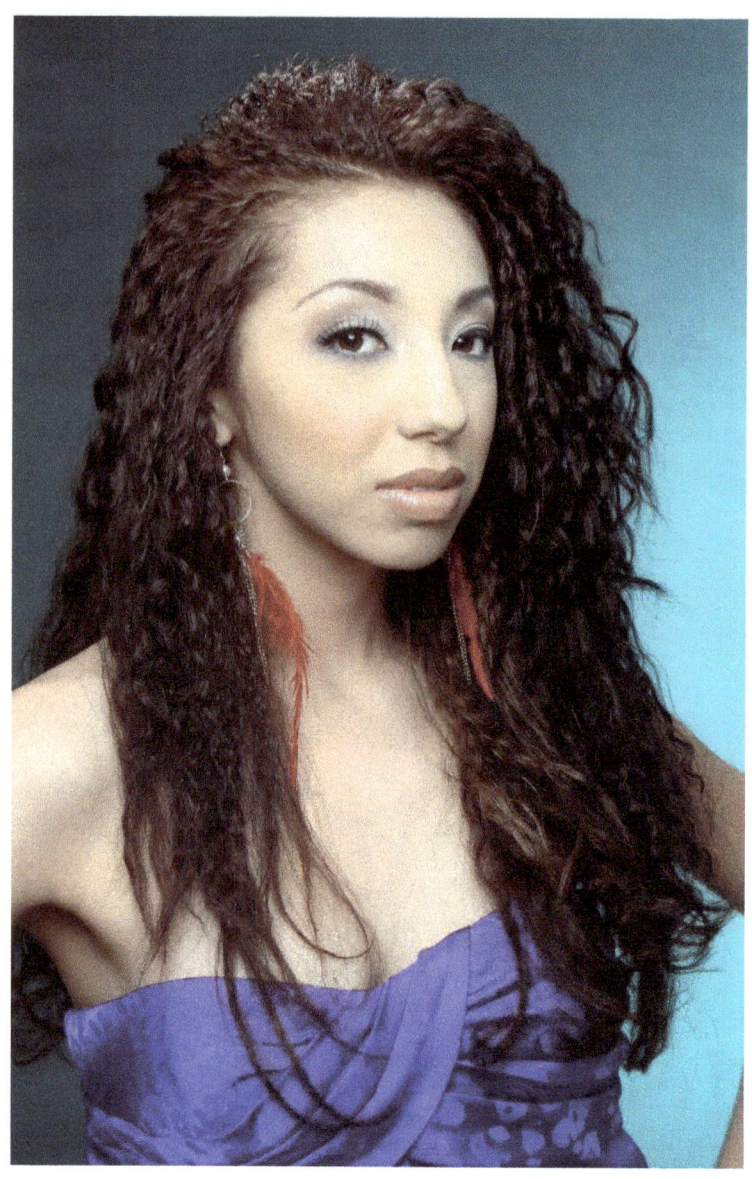

This technique adds texture and flexibility to straight hair, allowing you to be more creative.

Flexi-Rod Set Technique

Supplies: 4 butterfly clips, 4 duck bill clips, styling comb, rattail comb, 20-30 green flexi-rods, moisturizer, leave-in conditioner

Step 1: Apply moisturizer to clean hair.

Step 2: Apply leave-in conditioner.

Step 3: Section the hair into four sections using the butterfly clips.

Step 4: Start in the back of head separating small sections with the duck bill clips.

Step 5: Rod the hair by wrapping the hair around the rod.

Step 6: Repeat steps 4 through 5 until the whole head is completely in rods.

Step 7: Sit under hair dryer for 1 to 2 hours or until hair is dry.

Step 8: Unravel hair from the rods and style as desired.

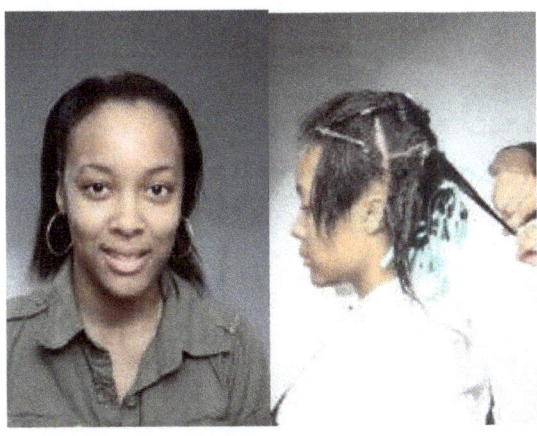

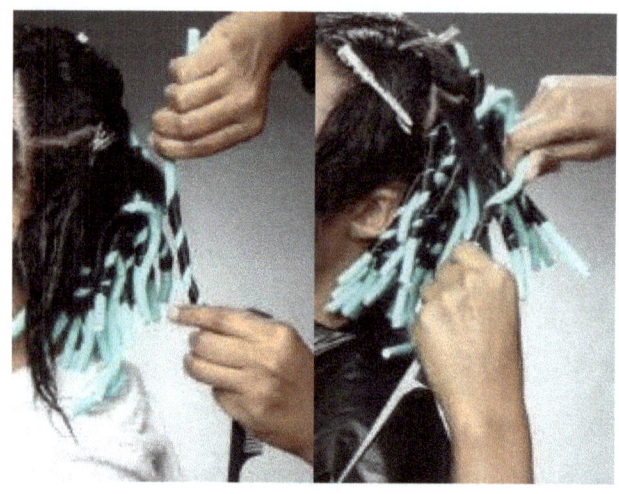

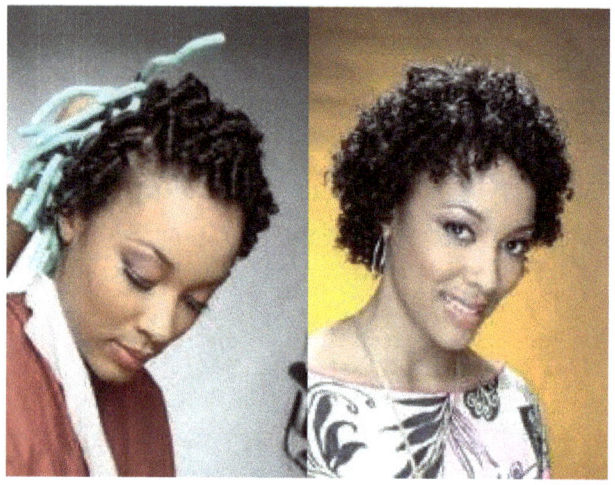

This style will create a textured look while adding shape and flexibility to any style.

"Protective styles are styles that are best for the condition of your hair."

Tiffany Anderson

It Takes One to Know One

I have shared and expressed my opinion openly in this book, and I feel like if I'm going to tell it, I should tell it all. I have been critical to the behaviors that we as black women have adapted to when we are trying to recreate unnatural images because of my own struggle with superficial gratification. This comes from my own personal experience and discovery of how I had been programmed to believe what beauty is. I experimented on myself trying to recreate what GOD had already made beautiful. I tried to perfect perfection. Whenever I would look in the mirror I would find something else wrong with the way I looked. I didn't like what I saw, not because of how I looked, but because of who I was. I did not feel like a beautiful black girl. I needed *Hair Therapy* bad. I had an unpolished feeling, and I believed that if I looked a certain way, I would be treated differently—better. Not realizing that it's not how you look or wear your hair but what you stand. Erroneously, I started to fall in love with how I *wanted* to look and not myself, which is a dangerous space to be in. That negative space was so close to me, reminding me daily of how I did not want to feel. I can remember wearing braids and still relaxing the edges of my hair, afraid of showing any curls because I thought people would know that my life wasn't smooth just as my hair wasn't smooth. I thought in order to make it seem as if I had a smooth life, I had to have smooth edges on my hair. I went out of my way investing in my hair and not in my business, as if my hair would take me further than my business. As I was doing all of these things, I realized I was a victim. A victim of low self-esteem! I needed unrealistic things to make me feel complete because I didn't feel complete without them. When I acknowledged this about myself, my journey and my purpose became clear. It is to share with women how to appreciate and take care of their crown and glory so they will not have to search for their beauty in other people's eyes. They can and will believe in their beauty from start to finish. When you love yourself you can embrace the beautiful black girl and not run away from her. It feels good to know that I don't need someone else's hair to compliment my look. I do not need cosmetic surgery to be proud of my body. I do not want to hide behind the variety of styles I have worn like it will make my past disappear. I want to embrace my own ignorance, remove my flaws, and channel my insecurities with freedom.

Please Don't

- Please don't shampoo your hair without conditioning it.
- Please don't substitute water for moisture.
- Please don't use water to re-wet the hair.
- Please don't use glue on the hair.
- Please don't use excessive tension on the hair.
- Please don't use box store products on the hair.
- Please don't comb out the hair without sectioning it.
- Please don't relax the hair.
- Please don't use rubber bands on the hair.
- Please don't use color on the hair without getting a skin test.
- Please don't wash the hair more than once a month.
- Please don't use oil for moisture.
- Please don't use excessive heat on the hair.

- Please don't leave styles up for more than the recommended time.
- Please don't use grease when pressing the hair.
- Please don't wet the hair every day.

Please Do

- Please do consult with a hair care professional (trichologist, natural hair expert, etc.).
- Please do read the ingredients in the products before use.
- Please do use a moisturizer.
- Please do wear a satin or silk sleep cap or scarf.
- Please do wear a shower cap.
- Please do use a wide tooth comb.
- Please do section the hair before combing the hair out.
- Please do use a moisturizer
- Please do stimulate the scalp.
- Please do consider the please don'ts before doing your hair.

Glossary

Alopecia- The partial or complete absence of hair from areas of the body where it normally grows; baldness.

Alopecia Areata- A type of hair loss that occurs when your immune system mistakenly attacks hair follicles, which is where hair growth begins. The damage to the follicle is usually not permanent. Experts do not know why the immune system attacks the follicles.

Braid- A length of hair made up of three or more interlaced strands.

Chemical- A compound or substance that has been purified or prepared, especially artificial.

Coarse- Rough or loose in texture or grain.

Cornrows- A style of braiding and plaiting the hair in narrow strips to form geometric patterns on the scalp.

Curly- Made, growing, or arranged in curls or curves.

DHT- Dihydrotestosterone is an endogenous androgen sex steroid and hormone.

Dry- Free from moisture or liquid; not wet or moist.

Female Pattern Baldness- Progressive loss of scalp hair in women, characterized by diffuse thinning on the crown but rarely leading to baldness; androgenetic alopecia.

Fine- Thin, light, delicate, wispy, flyaway.

Hair- Hairs collectively, especially those growing on a person's head.

Male Pattern Baldness- Related to genes and male sex hormones (dihydrotestosterone). It usually follows a pattern of receding hairline and hair thinning on the crown, and is caused by hormones and genetic predisposition.

Moisture- Water or other liquid diffused in a small quantity as vapor, within a solid, condensed on a surface.

Natural- Existing in or caused by raised nature; not made or caused by humankind.

Relaxed Hair- A relaxer is a type of lotion or cream generally used by people with tight curls or very curly which makes hair easier to straighten by chemically relaxing the natural curls. The active agent is usually a strong alkali, although some formulations are based on ammonium thioglycolate instead.

Senegalese Twist- Dividing the hairs into several sections, twisting strands of hair, then twisting two twisted strands around one another.

Technique – a skillful or efficient way of doing or achieving something.

Texture- Give a rough or texture.

Traction Alopecia- Is a form of alopecia or gradual hair loss, caused primarily by pulling force being applied to the hair. This commonly results from the sufferer frequently wearing their hair in a particularly tight ponytail, pigtails, or braids.

Trichologist- The branch of medical and cosmetic study and practice concerned with the hair and scalp.

Twist- A thing with a spiral shape.

Virgin Hair- Hair that is completely unprocessed and intact. To qualify as virgin hair, it must meet rigorous standards including: not been permed, dyed, colored, bleached, or chemically processed in any way.

* * * * * *

FORWARD

Natural hair is most beautiful when it is appreciated and shared. As women, we owe it to ourselves to give and to pass on information from one generation to the next. This book would not be complete if we did not help our baby naturals become confident adult naturals. To be successful with a message we must understand that it must be embedded.

I have created a natural hair section for kids. This section is an introduction to a young natural that will help little girl's beginning their natural hair movement. They will understand the importance of caring for their hair. After reading "I Love My Natural Hair" your little natural will pride herself and ask questions that will motivate a parent to want to be more creative with styles and techniques. This book will entertain as well as inspire with a fresh, fun, humorous collection of pros that deal with a subject that isn't always fun and humorous. Her first Natural hair book.

I ♥ My Natural Hair

Tiffany Anderson
Illustrated by Kenny Martin Jr.

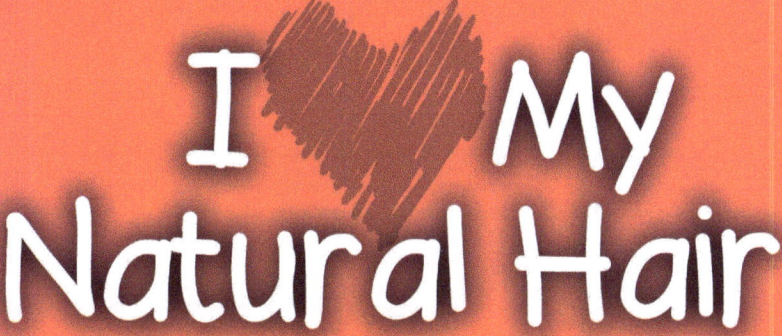

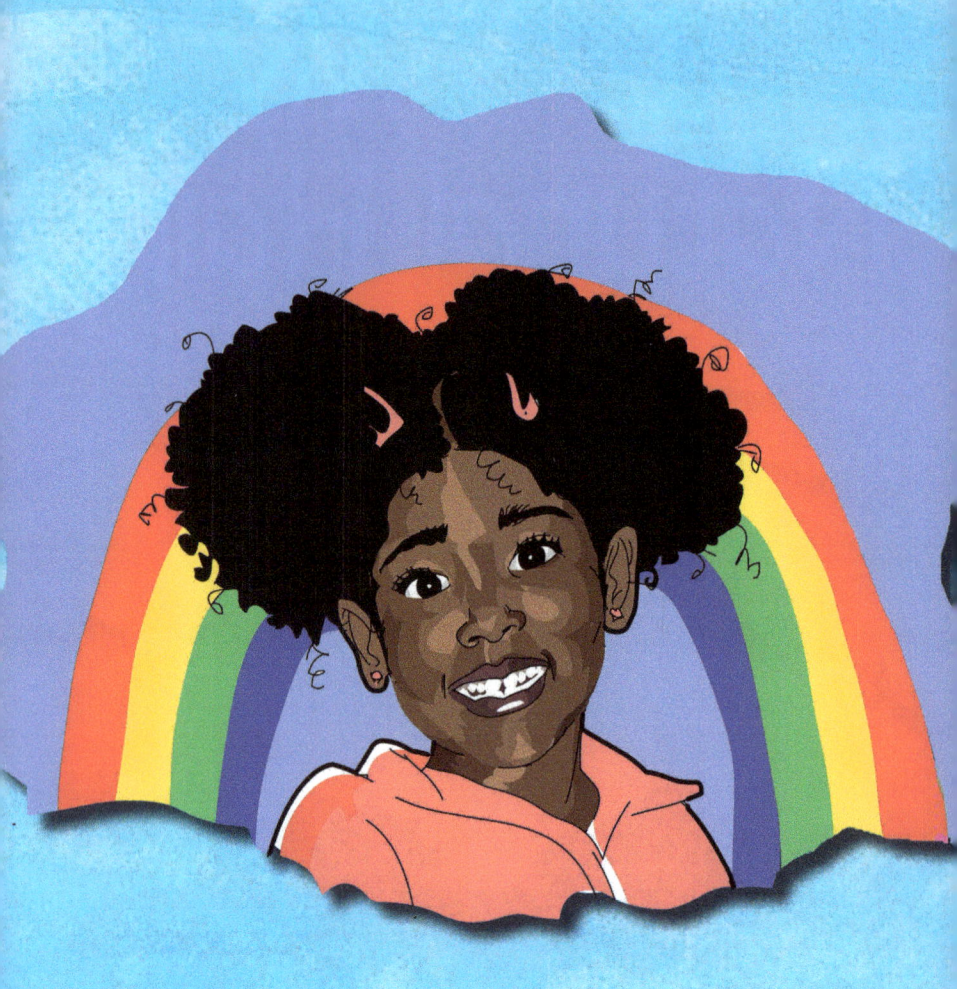

I love my natural hair because it can be curly...

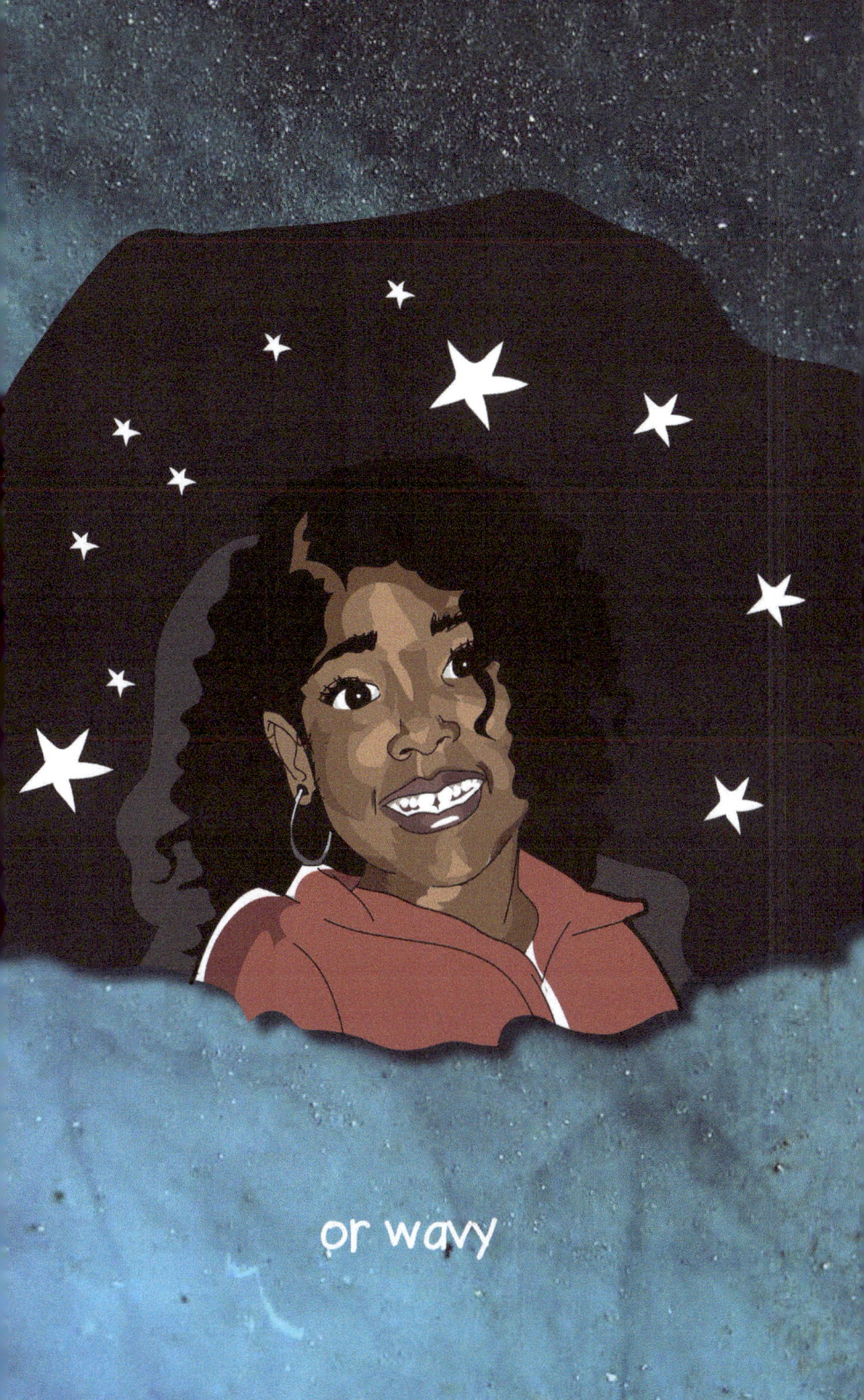

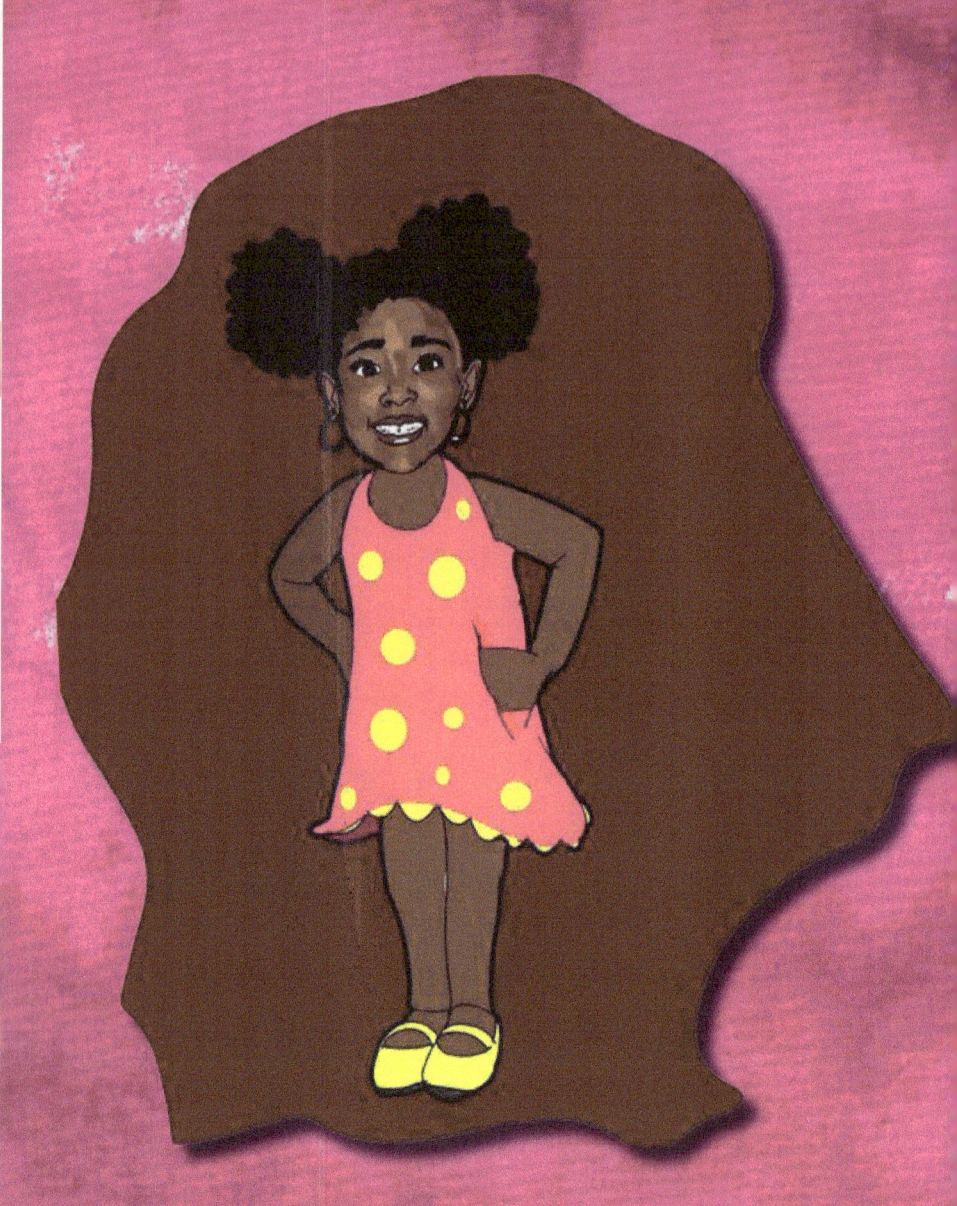

I love my natural hair because it's a part of me

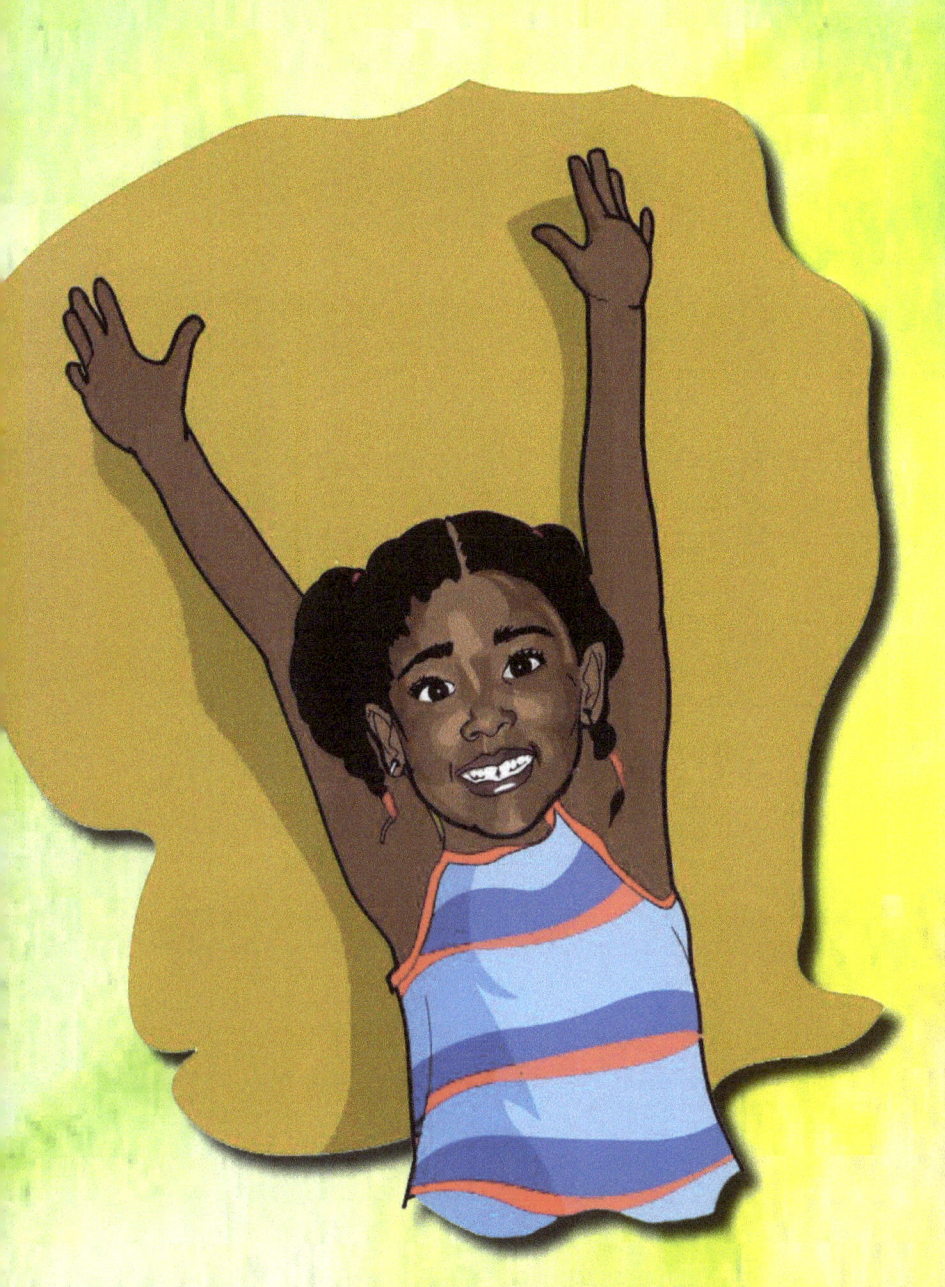

Some may think that natural isn't the best way to be

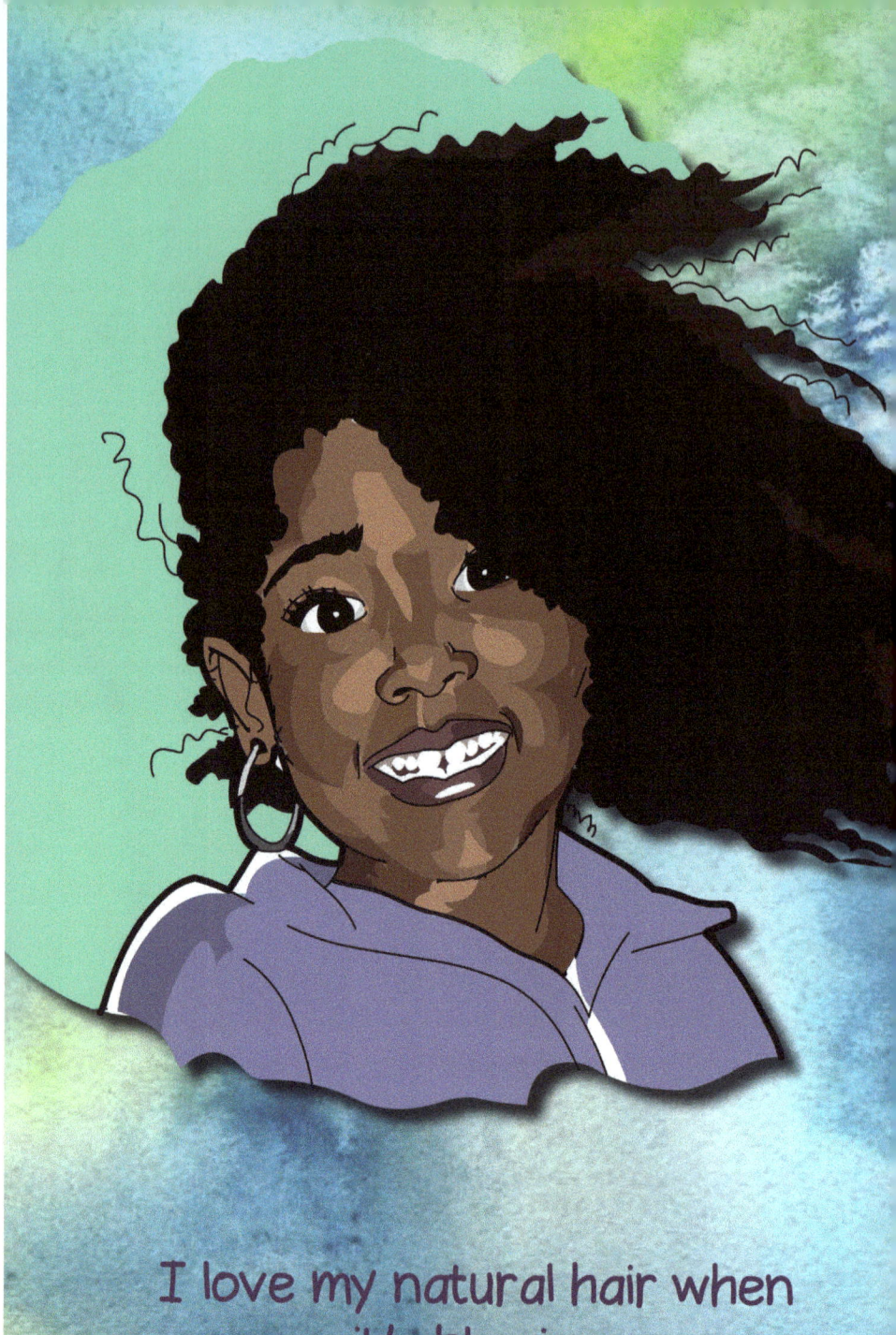

I love my natural hair when it's blowing

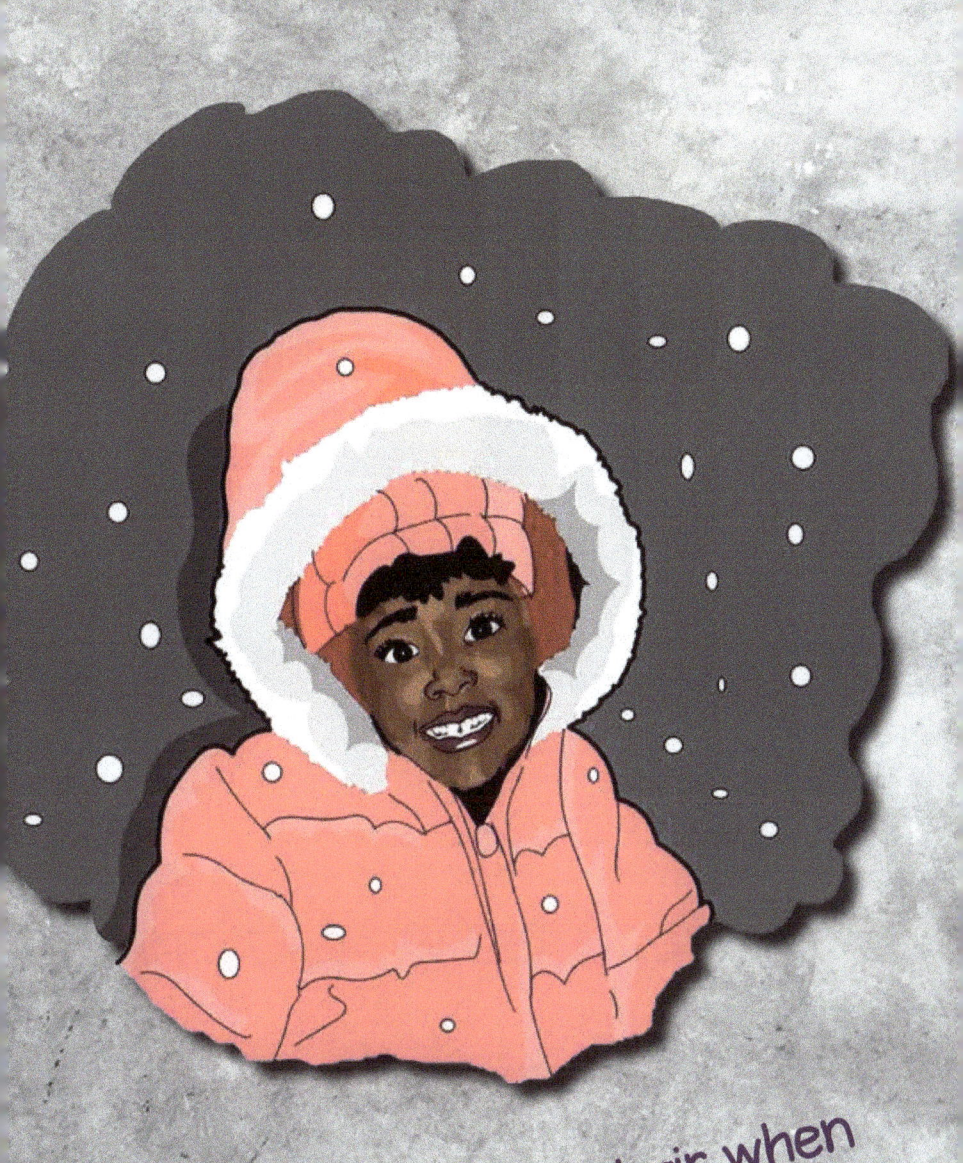

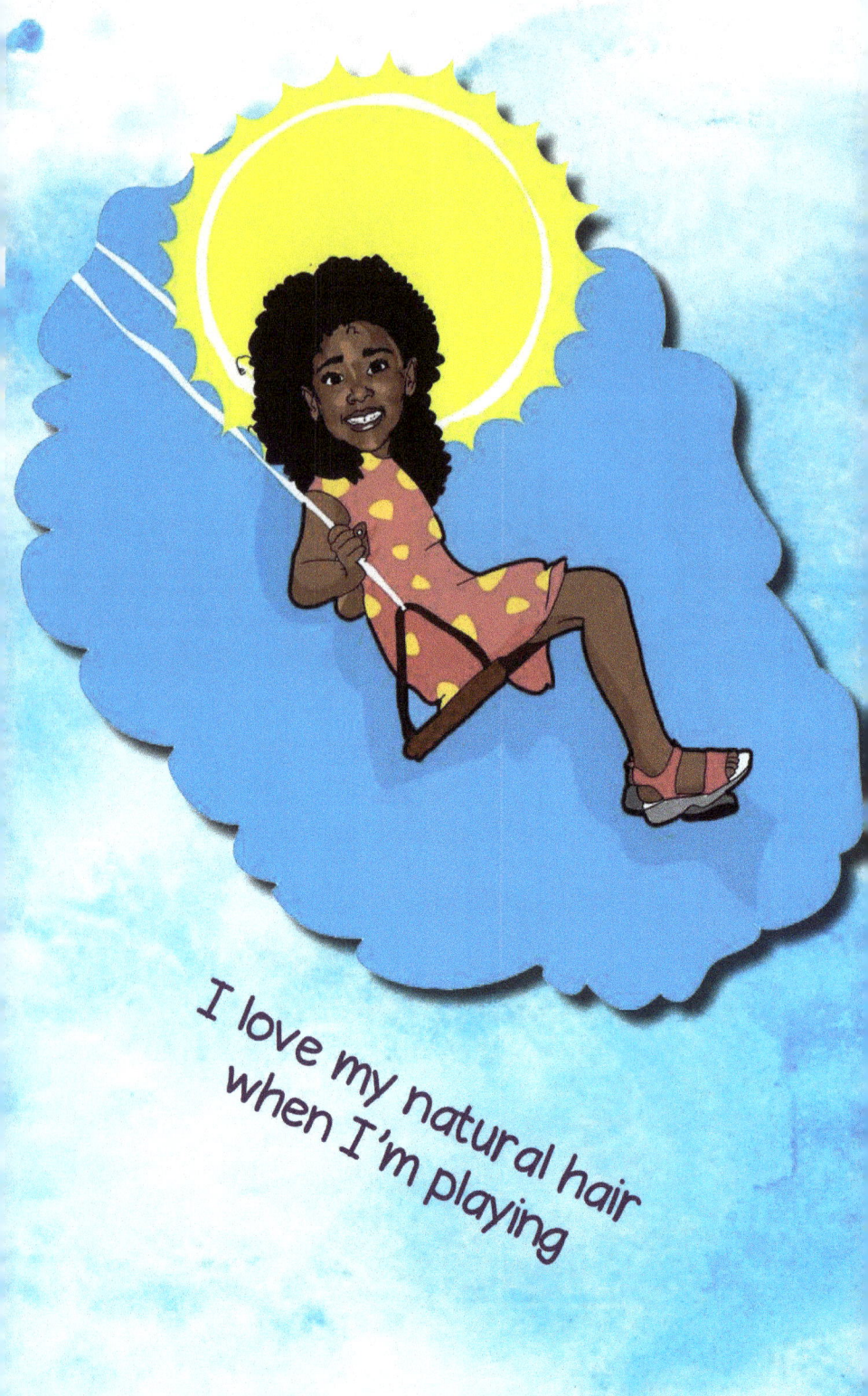

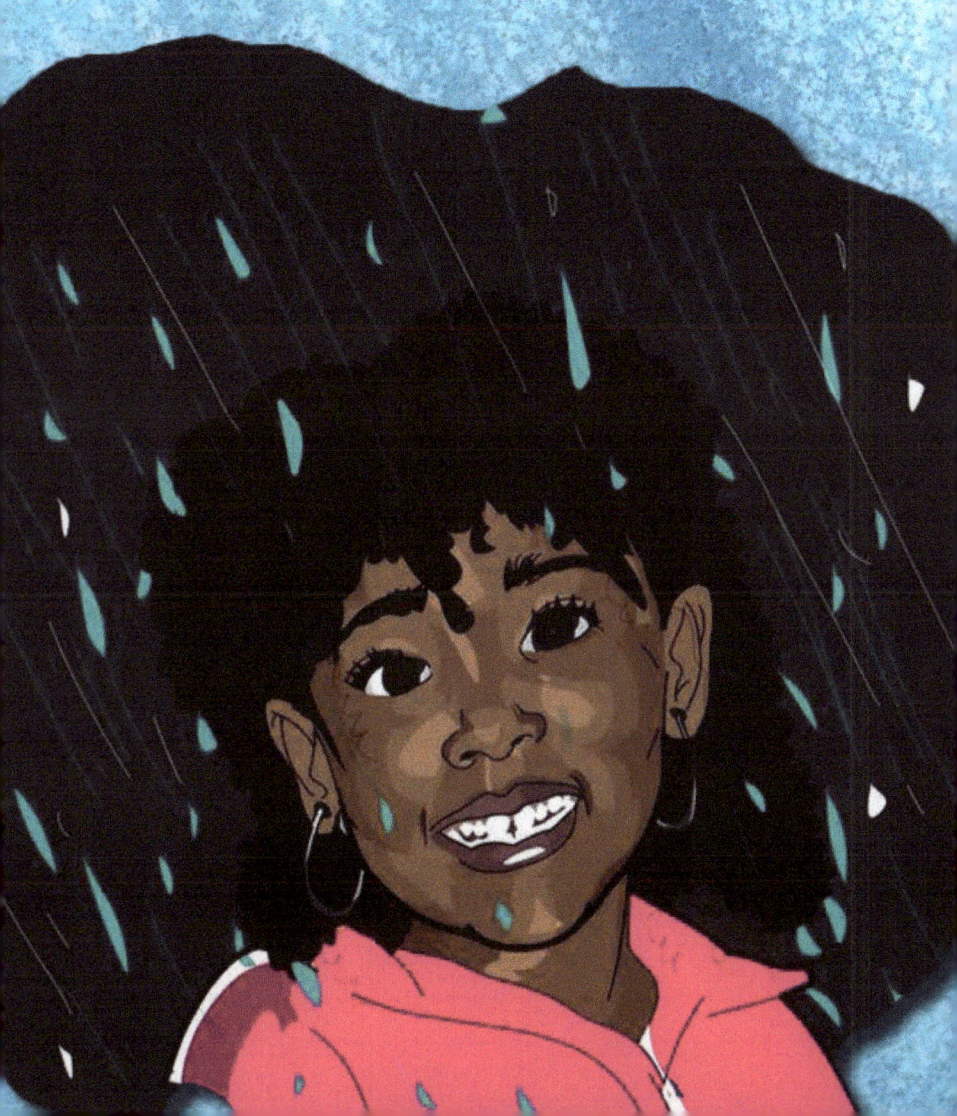

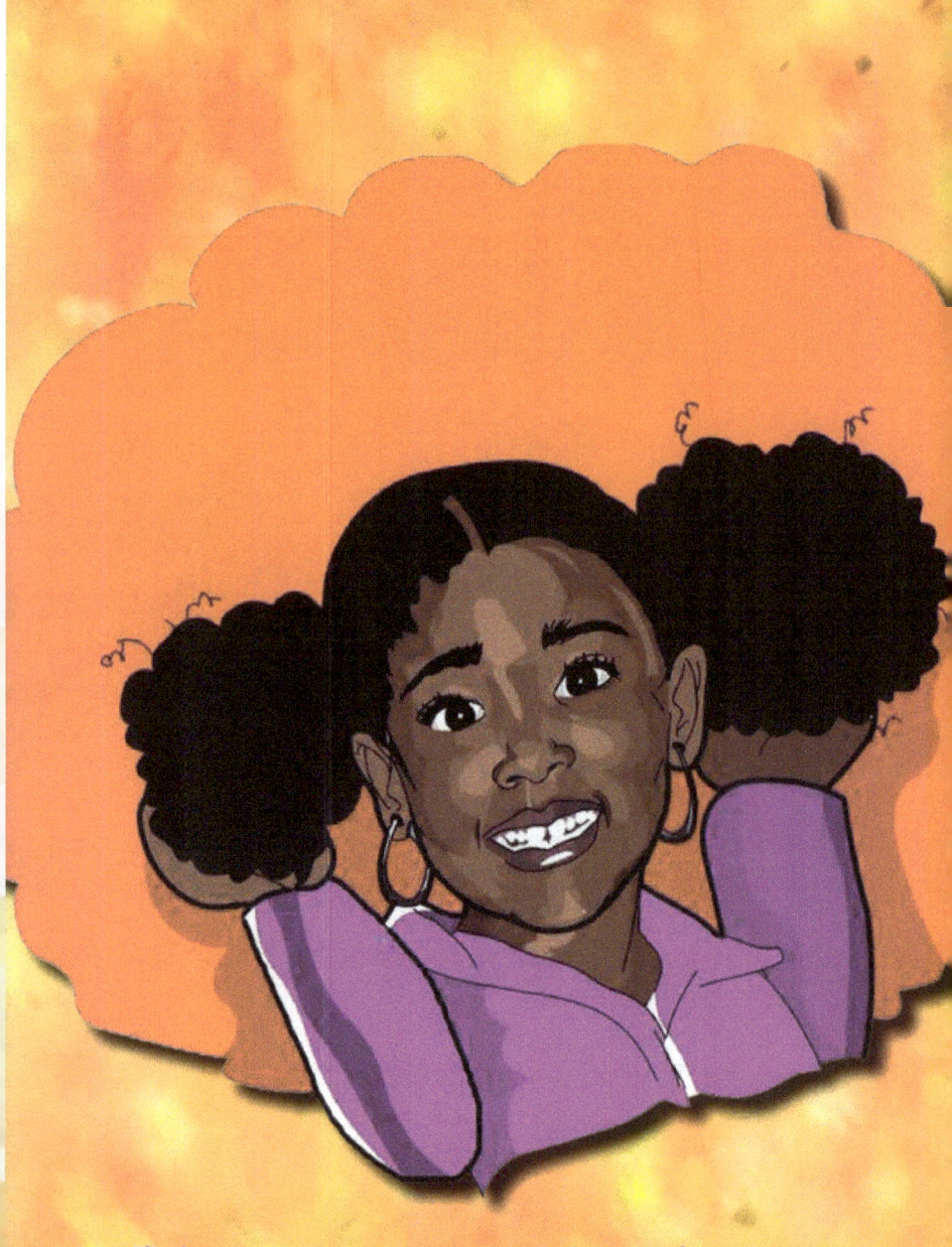

I love my natural hair because it's healthy and strong

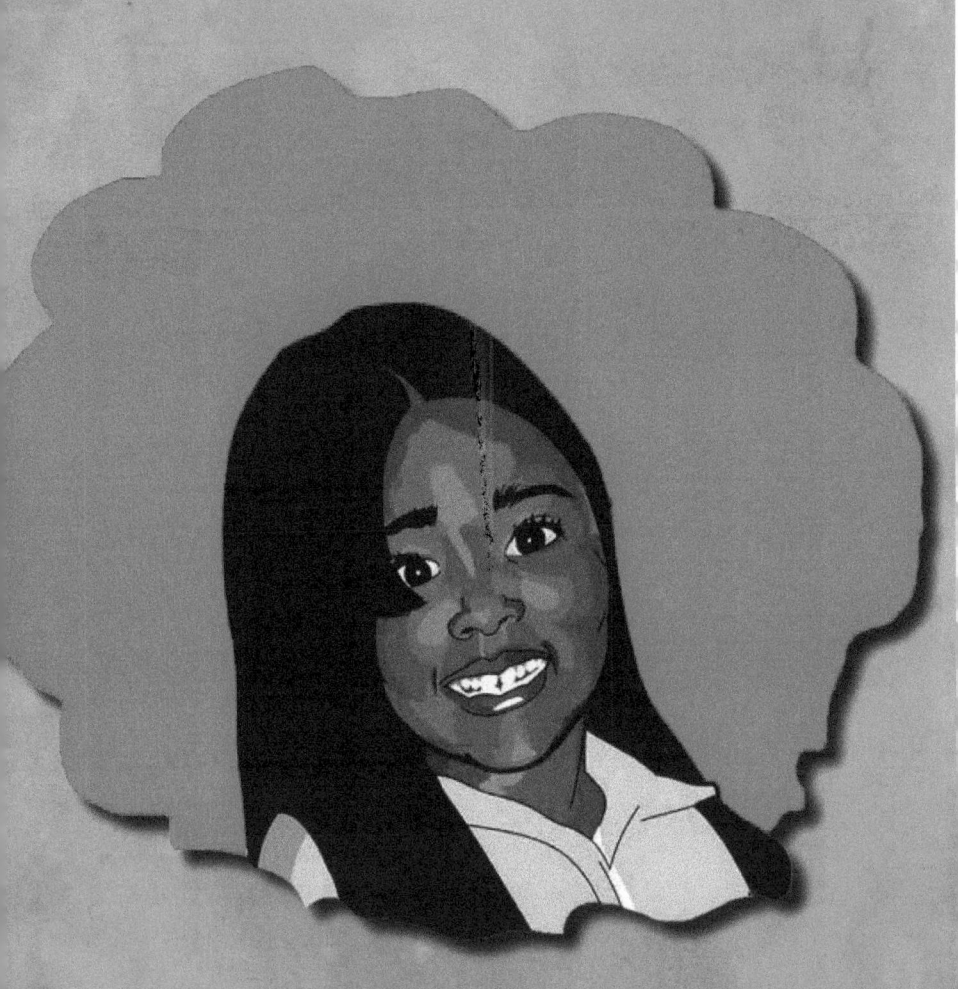

or long

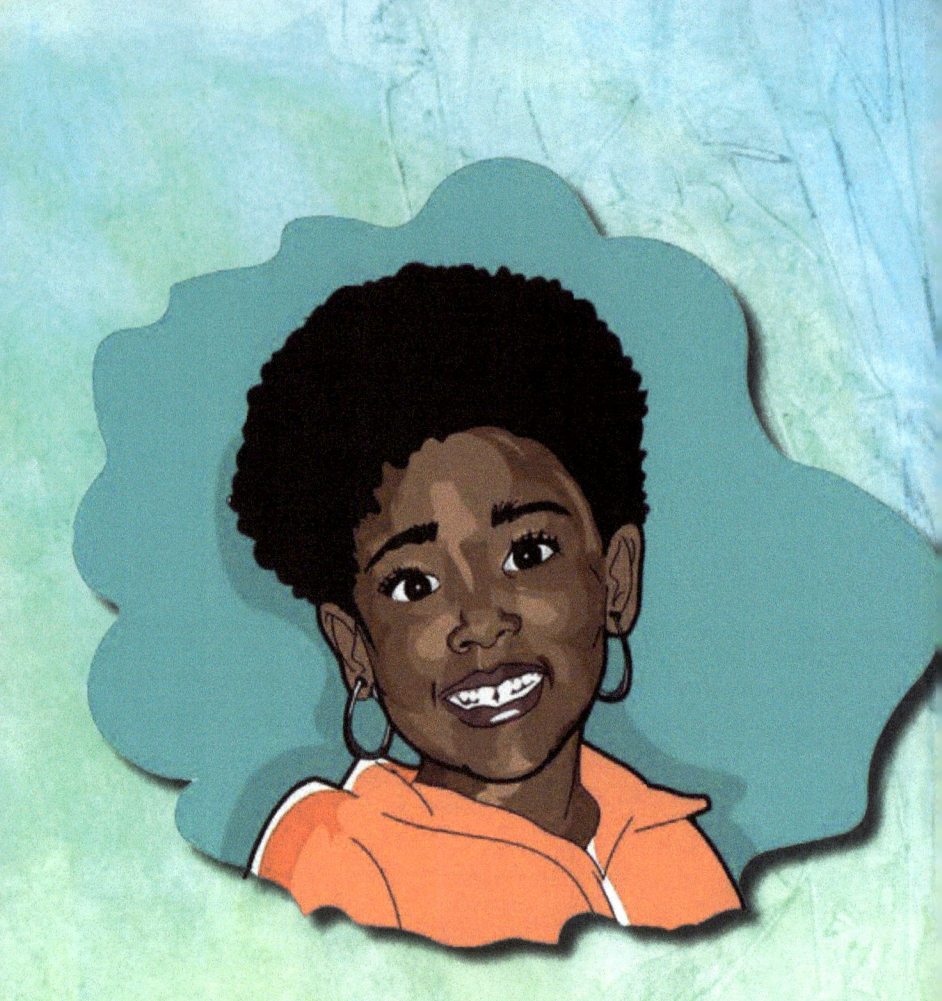

I love my natural hair because it can be short

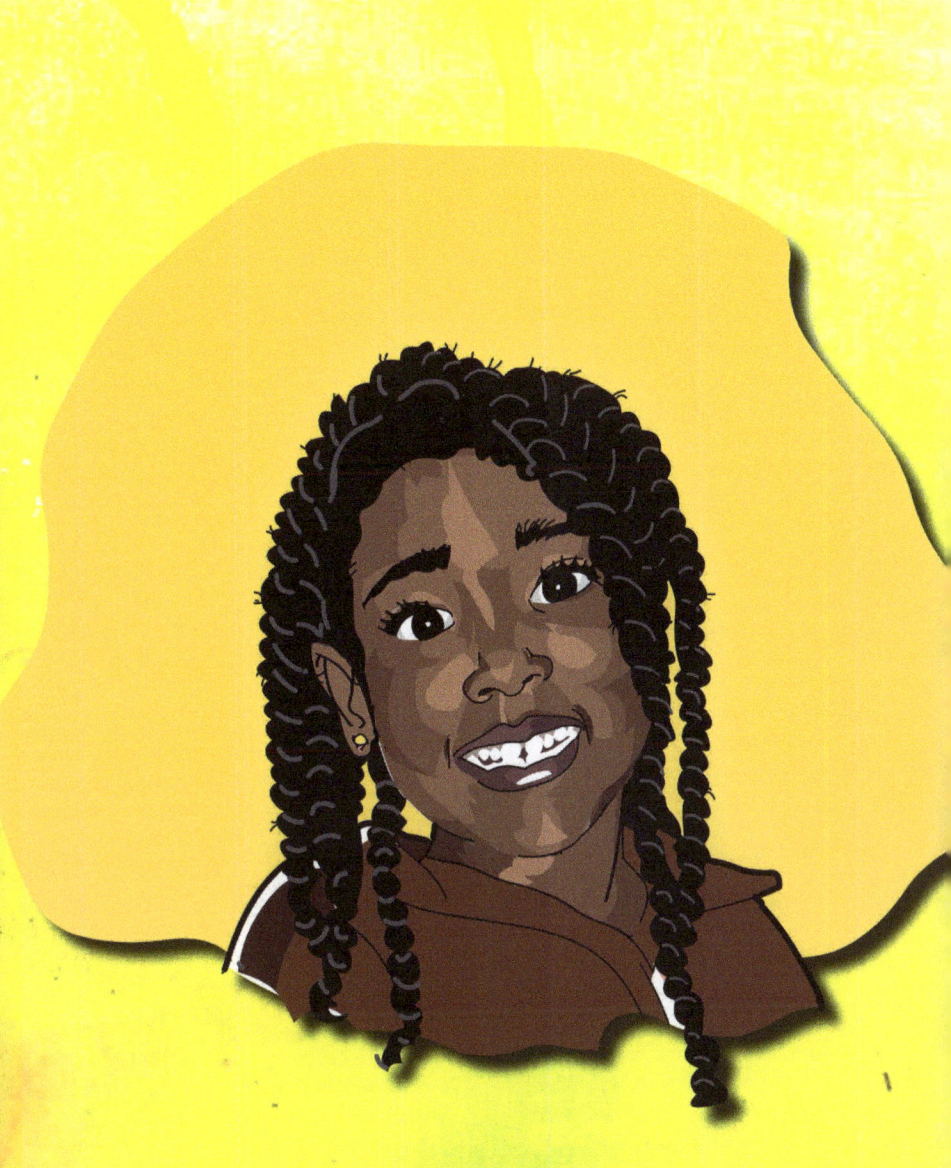

or twisted

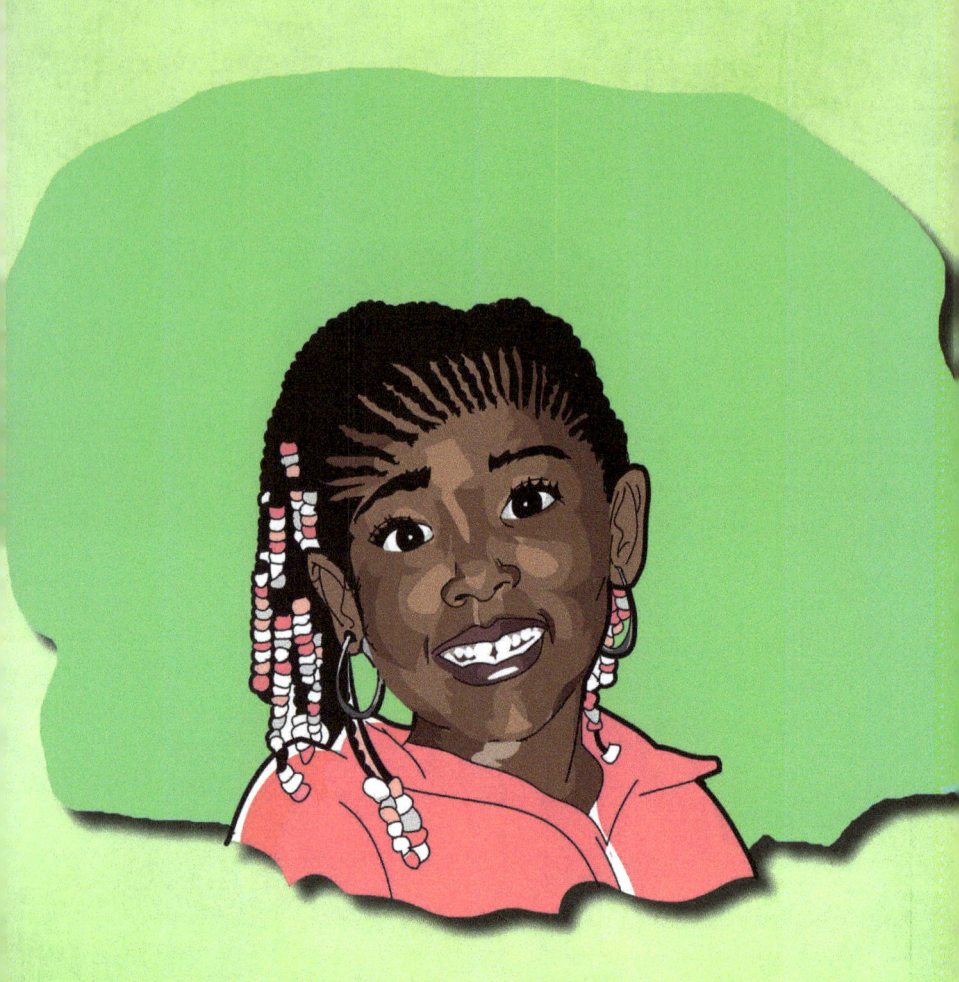

braided

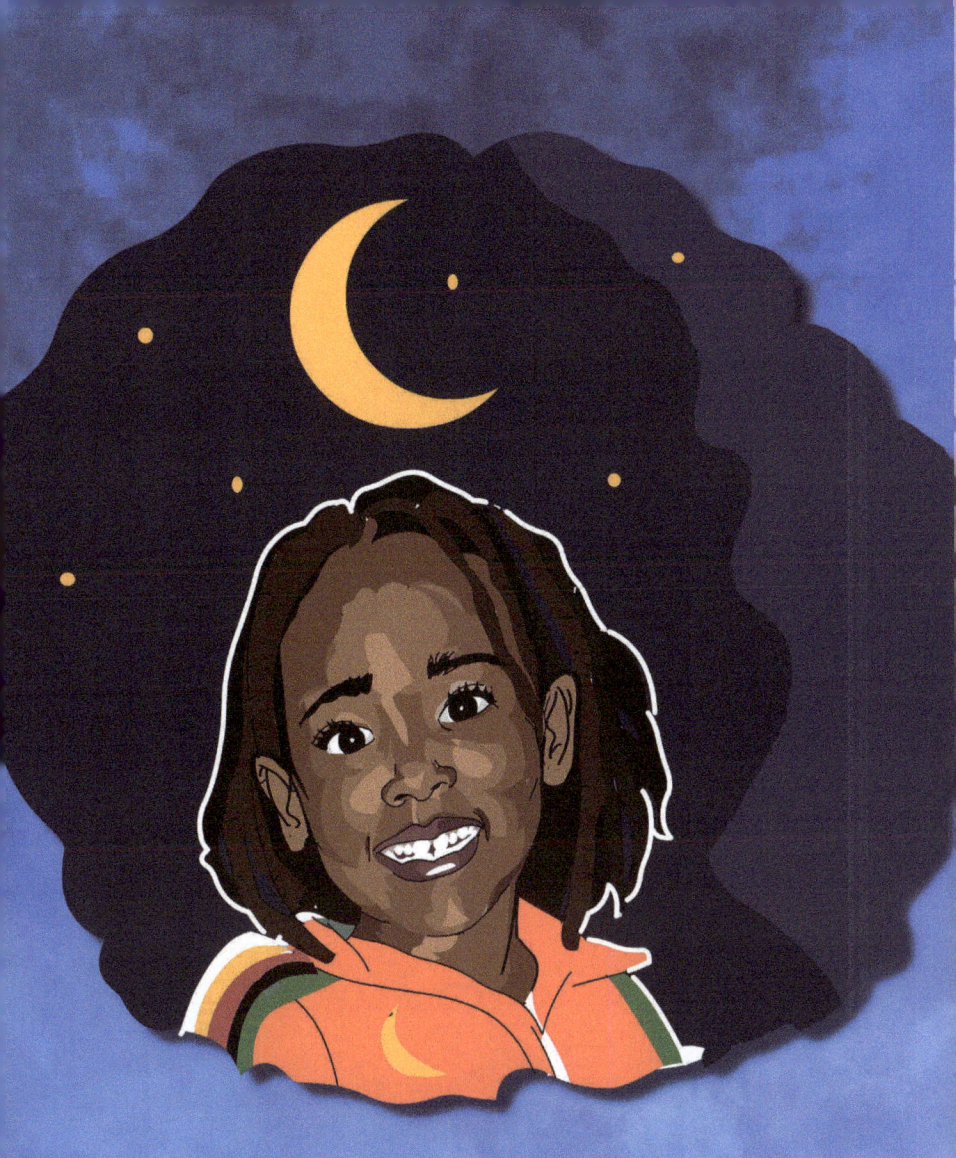

I love my natural hair because it can be locked

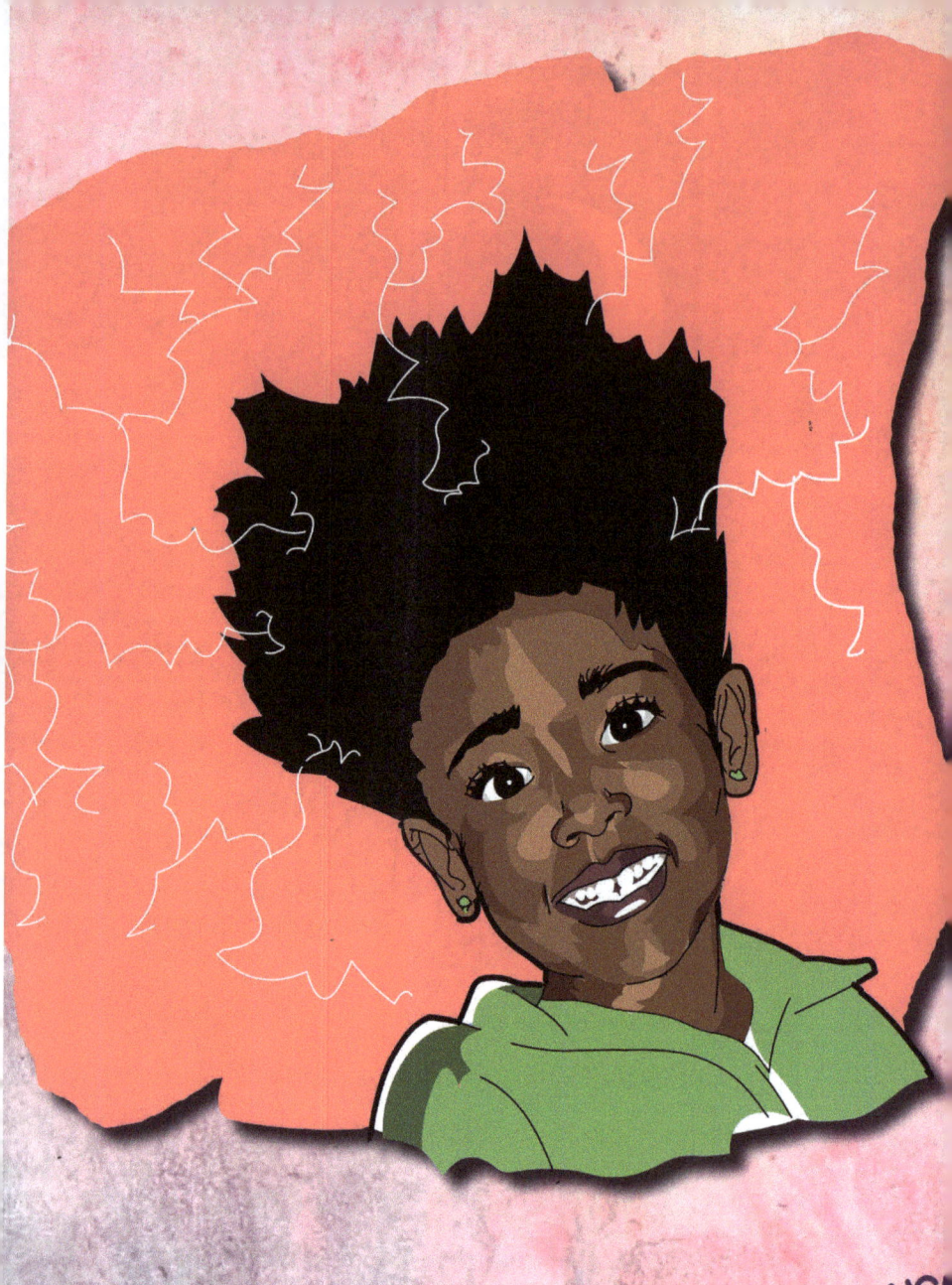

www.ingramcontent.com/pod-product-compliance
Ingram Content Group UK Ltd.
Pitfield, Milton Keynes, MK11 3LW, UK
UKHW021253180426
11947UKWH00010B/761